The DECLINE of THERAPEUTIC BLOODLETTING

and the Collapse of Traditional Medicine

The DECLINE of THERAPEUTIC BLOODLETTING

and the
Collapse
of
Traditional
Medicine

K. CODELL CARTER

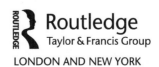

Routledge
Taylor & Francis Group

LONDON AND NEW YORK

First published 2012 by Transaction Publishers

2 Park Square, Milton Park, Abingdon, Oxfordshire OX14 4RN
711 Third Avenue, New York, NY 10017

Routledge is an imprint of the Taylor & Francis Group, an informa business

First issued in paperback 2017

Library of Congress Catalog Number: 2011042475

Library of Congress Cataloging-in-Publication Data

Carter, K. Codell (Kay Codell), 1939–
  The decline of therapeutic bloodletting and the collapse of traditional medicine / K. Codell Carter.
       p. cm.
  Includes bibliographical references and index.
  ISBN 978-1-4128-4604-2 (alk. paper)
  I. Title.
  [DNLM: 1. Bloodletting—history—Europe.   2. Attitude to Health—Europe.   3. History, 19th Century—Europe.   4. Medicine, Traditional—history—Europe.   WB 381]
       615.8′8—dc23

                                                              2011042475

ISBN 13: 978-1-4128-4604-2 (hbk)
ISBN 13: 978-1-138-51568-0 (pbk)

Contents

Preface

I have been working on this book for most of my professional career, and much of it draws on my earlier publications. These earlier works can be seen as preliminary studies for this volume. This book is intended to take a broad view, and so it is impossible to fully develop and defend all of the claims I will here advance. Many such claims are more fully documented in the cited preliminary studies that preceded this volume.

The immediate incentive for the completion of this book is David Wootton's *Bad Medicine: Doctors Doing Harm Since Hippocrates*, which I first discovered in 2010. Wootton's book focuses heavily on the practical, therapeutic side of medicine, and in my opinion, it does not begin to do justice to the theoretical innovations on which scientific medicine (including modern therapy) depend. Indeed, Wootton himself observes that while, in developing scientific medicine, "There were conceptual obstacles to be overcome, . . . it is difficult to see that those obstacles were major ones" (p. 284). In fact, the obstacles were enormous—arguably greater than the conceptual obstacles in moving from a geocentric to a heliocentric interpretation of the apparent motion of the heavens. The rise of modern medicine involved not just a change in how diseases and disease causation were to be conceived (a theoretical change more or less parallel to changes in the reference point for describing the heavenly motion), but a change in the role that the vast institution of medicine was to play in society. Because he underestimates the magnitude of this problem, Wootton raises several important questions that he is unable to answer. To take one prominent example, he astutely observes that the collapse of traditional medicine was a *precondition* for the rise of modern medicine, but he gives no support for this insightful claim—a claim that can be understood only by taking account of the theoretical innovations on which scientific medicine depends. So this deficiency can be traced to Wootton's failure to grasp the crucial conceptual (one might even say, philosophical) innovations that were required before traditional medicine could be overthrown and modern scientific medicine could begin.

In *The Rise of Causal Concepts of Disease*, I gave extensive attention to the theoretical side of medicine, and I largely ignored therapy. Yet, all along, I have been very much interested in the collapse of bloodletting. Ever since my first publication on the topic (1982), I realized that the relation between the decline of the traditional therapies and the rise of scientific medicine was not at all what one might have expected, and I have intended to write a book exploring this relation. I am very much indebted to David Wootton, not least for providing me with the incentive, finally, to bring this project to completion. I must also thank the editors of several journals and publishers for permission to use materials from earlier published essays. These include the following: parts of chapter 1 draw heavily on "Leechcraft in Nineteenth Century British Medicine" from the *Journal of the Royal Society of Medicine*, much of chapter 2 was published as "On the Decline of Bloodletting in Nineteenth Century Medicine" in *The Journal of Psychoanalytic Anthropology*, a good part of chapter 3 is adapted from the chapter entitled "Causes of Disease in Early Nineteenth-century Practical Medicine" that appeared in *The Rise of Causal Concepts of Disease* (published by Ashgate Publishing Company), chapter 4 is adapted from "The Concept of Quackery in Early Nineteenth Century British Medical Periodicals" published in *The Journal of Medical Humanities*, chapter 5 is adapted from "Change of Type as an Explanation for the Decline of Therapeutic Bloodletting" from *Studies in the History and Philosophy of the Biological and Biomedical Sciences*, parts of chapter 6 resemble parts of many of my earlier publications on Ignaz Semmelweis but, most closely, perhaps, the chapter entitled "Etiological Characterizations" from *Rise of Causal Concepts of Disease* (Ashgate Publishing Company) and parts of *Childbed Fever: A Scientific Biography of Ignaz Semmelweis* (published by Greenwood Press and by Transaction Publishers). Some of the ideas in chapter 7 are based on the chapter entitled "A Bacterial Theory of Disease" from *Rise of Causal Concepts of Disease* (Ashgate Publishing Company) and on "Early Conjectures that Down Syndrome is Caused by Chromosomal Nondisjunction" from *Bulletin of the History of Medicine*. Full bibliographic details for all of these publications can be found in the list of references at the end of this volume. Most of the materials from these earlier publications have been rewritten and reorganized, and my analysis has been considerably expanded throughout.

I must also thank innumerable students most of whom have found it fun and worthwhile to learn about bloodletting and causal thinking in medicine. I am grateful to Brigham Young University for continued support and for providing a wonderful environment in which to study and learn. Most of all I thank my wife, Barbara, for her boundless confidence, her unflagging encouragement, and for lots of Salzburger Nockerl.

Introduction

Science never makes an advance until philosophy authorizes and directs it to do so.
—Thomas Mann, *"Freud und die Zukunft" (1936)*

The decline of therapeutic bloodletting is among the most curious developments in all of social or scientific history. Bloodletting was the most prominent medical therapy in early nineteenth-century Europe. From there, it can be traced back, without interruption, to Greek and Roman physicians many of whom regarded it as among their most important and successful therapies. The Hippocratic corpus contains numerous discussions of bloodletting. Galen, certainly the most famous physician in classical antiquity, wrote tracts explaining and defending the practice. It was employed in ancient Egypt and is the most commonly mentioned therapy in the Babylonian Talmud (Carter, 1991). Indeed, it was practiced in virtually every part of the ancient world; it was prominent in the classical medical systems of India and China (from whence, almost certainly, arose what we now know as acupuncture [Epler, 1980]). It was (and in some cases still is) practiced among the indigenous peoples of Africa, South-East Asia, Pacific Islands, Amazon basin, and North America. Then, in nineteenth-century Europe, over the course of about a single generation, without significant discussion or debate, it was almost completely abandoned. Even while this was happening, almost no one seemed to have argued against the practice or to have provided any reason to believe that it was ineffective. Indeed, no such reasons could have been given because *bloodletting actually worked*; it really did accomplish exactly what it was intended to accomplish, and contemporary physicians—the very ones who gave it up—were fully aware of this fact. In 1856, one Scottish

1

physician observed that the discussion of the merits of bloodletting *followed* rather than *preceded* its abandonment and that the physicians who, in his day, were advocating its use were the very practitioners who acknowledged having given it up (Bennett, 1856–7b). How is all of this to be explained?

Nowadays, therapeutic bloodletting, and, indeed, the entire medical system to which it was central, is generally deemed to have been ineffective or even positively harmful. Bloodletting is sometimes dismissed as yet another bizarre and inexplicable quirk of human behavior—something on a par with cannibalism or self-flagellation. Joseph Agassi, a philosopher of science, denounced bloodletting as "the single greatest error in the history of medicine" and claimed that only after it was abandoned "did doctors start doing more good than harm" (Agassi, 1969, p. 5). The American sociologist Lawrence J. Henderson was similarly skeptical of the therapies of traditional medicine; he concluded that not until somewhere between 1910 and 1920, did a random patient, with a random disease, consulting a doctor chosen at random, have, for the first time in the history of mankind, a better than fifty–fifty chance of profiting from the encounter (quoted in Conrad and Schneider, 1980, p. 33). In his recent book, *Bad Medicine: Doctors Doing Harm Since Hippocrates*, David Wootton advances a similar position: "If we define medicine as the ability to cure diseases, then there was very little medicine before 1865. The long tradition that descended from Hippocrates, symbolized by a reliance on bloodletting, purges, and emetics, was almost totally ineffectual, indeed positively deleterious, except in so far as it mobilized the placebo effect" (Wootton, 2007, p. 283). But surely it would be astonishing if, for *millennia*, in spite of their best efforts and good intentions, tens of thousands of intelligent and dedicated physicians simply got it all wrong. And, in striking contrast to these modern critics, nineteenth-century physicians were absolutely certain that bloodletting was effective: "whatever explanation may be given of the effects of bloodletting, there is no doubt of its multiplied results in the treatment of disease" (Wardrop, 1833). So who are we to believe? Was bloodletting simply a colossal mistake? Or was it truly effective in some way, and if so, how?

However, if early nineteenth-century physicians were so convinced that bloodletting worked, why was the practice suddenly abandoned? It is tempting to assume that such a profound change must have resulted from some kind of scientific discovery or carefully reasoned argument, and on the basis of this assumption, some historians have seized on two publications by the French physician Pierre-Charles-Alexandre Louis. In 1828, Louis published a paper entitled "Research on the effects of bloodletting in some inflammatory diseases" (Louis, 1828). Seven years later, in 1835, an expanded and slightly revised version of the paper appeared as a short book; in 1836, this book was translated into English. Louis's two publications are sometimes proclaimed as the first scientific challenge to bloodletting. This view goes back at least as far as Erwin Ackerknecht's monumental 1946 *History of Medicine* (Ackerknecht, 1946, p. 134), and, even now, at the time of this writing, this view continues to appear in that famous and unimpeachable source of conventional wisdom, Wikipedia. But while Louis's conclusions are not entirely unambiguous, he himself interpreted his results as *supporting* (rather than as challenging) the timely use of bloodletting, and, in the 1850s, his publications were seldom mentioned in extensive discussions of why bloodletting had been abandoned. So it is far from clear that Louis can be seen as a serious opponent of bloodletting or that his work significantly eroded confidence in the practice. But otherwise, no early nineteenth-century publications have been identified that contained arguments against therapeutic bloodletting—no serious objections seem ever to have been raised against the practice; certainly, there were none until well after it was already in decline.

However, if bloodletting was not refuted by any direct scientific argument, why was it given up at all? Surely it cannot be a simple coincidence that scientific medicine arose approximately at the same time that the traditional therapies were being abandoned; these two developments, so clearly related, must have had some influence on one another. So what, exactly, was the relation between the rise of scientific medicine and the decline of bloodletting? Suppose one takes the general medical acceptance of the germ theory of disease as a convenient marker for the beginning of what we now see as scientific medicine. Although there were obviously precursors and earlier contributors, what was probably the first articulation of the modern germ theory appeared in an 1875 publication by Edwin Klebs (Klebs, 1875–6), and, according to Louis Pasteur, the germ theory first became generally accepted by about the beginning of the 1880s, at about the time of the London International Medical Congress (Pasteur, 1881, p. 370). Yet, by 1850—approximately thirty years earlier—physicians already spoke of the therapeutic use of bloodletting as in sharp decline. So the collapse of what is sometimes called traditional or Hippocratic medicine, which included bloodletting as its most prominent therapy, *preceded* and so cannot have been a direct consequence of the general acceptance of scientific medicine.

David Wootton astutely and correctly observed that "the demise of Hippocratic medicine was a *precondition* for the triumph of germ theory" (Wootton, 2007, p. 143). But Wootton does not explain this important and insightful claim, and the only justification he provides is seriously inadequate. According to Wootton, in the 1820s, the therapies of traditional medicine—the most prominent of which was bloodletting—"began to be exposed as worthless," and this, supposedly, occasioned a sort of crisis and a frantic quest for new therapies (Wootton, 2007, p. 143). Wootton's view may reflect the reasonable (but entirely incorrect) *a priori* assumption that, before bloodletting could have been abandoned, it *must*, somehow, have been shown not to work. But Wootton provides no evidence in support of this claim and, in fact, nothing of the sort ever happened. Bloodletting was never exposed as worthless; there was never any evidence that it didn't work—there couldn't have been any such evidence because, as I have already observed, it really did accomplish exactly what it was intended to accomplish. Moreover, bloodletting was given up without any significant argument or debate, something that would have been almost unimaginable if this cherished and ancient therapy had somehow been under direct attack. And even if bloodletting had been proven worthless, that by itself would still not explain why the collapse of Hippocratic medicine was a *precondition* for the rise of the germ theory of disease—why, one might wonder, would it have been *impossible* for the germ theory to arise *before* the collapse of traditional medicine and thereby to have at least contributed to its decline? So what, exactly, was the relation between the collapse of the traditional therapies and the rise of modern medicine?

The process by which scientific medicine supplanted traditional medicine took a path quite different from what one might expect. In fact, what would usually be thought of as scientific considerations, for example, statistical studies or the accumulation of experimental evidence, had virtually nothing to do with overcoming the traditional therapies. Indeed, the collapse of traditional medicine was very definitely a precondition for the very beginning of scientific medicine—a precondition that had to be met, not just before the germ theory of disease could *triumph* (to use Wootton's term), but before that theory could even be *conceived of.* As currently formulated, the germ theory of disease would have been absolutely unthinkable given the conceptual framework of traditional medicine. The very concept of disease on which Hippocratic medicine rested had to be given up and an entirely new way of thinking adopted before the germ theory could even make sense. But, at least as science is often understood, this conceptual change was not, strictly speaking, a matter of science. In a sense, traditional medicine collapsed partly because of social changes and partly because of what might be called semantic or even philosophical considerations. Scientific medicine did not overthrow traditional medicine. It may be more accurate to say that science filled a void that was left by the collapse of the older system. So how, exactly, was the collapse of Hippocratic medicine a precondition for the rise of scientific medicine? And if the considerations that led to the collapse of traditional medicine were not strictly scientific, what, exactly, were they?

Curiously enough, the key to answering all of these questions is to be found in *leechcraft*, that is, in therapeutic bloodletting—the therapy that symbolized and virtually defined the practice of medicine at the beginning of the nineteenth century. Until one understands bloodletting, one cannot understand the system of medicine in which it was the central and defining therapy. If one doesn't understand this system of medicine, one cannot understand *either* what social benefits this system provided *or* why it ultimately collapsed. And if one cannot understand why traditional medicine collapsed, one cannot possibly explain how or why that collapse was a precondition for the rise of the germ theory. So we must begin by getting clear about bloodletting. Doing so will help us see the practice as something more than a colossal mistake, and it will help us understand how traditional medicine could have persisted so tenaciously for thousands of years all the while without having (what would today be seen as) significant therapeutic value; it will also help us discover why and in what sense the collapse of traditional medicine was, indeed, a true logical *precondition* for the rise of the germ theory of disease.

I must make clear, at the start, how I envision my current project. Several decades ago, the Hungarian philosopher Imre Lakatos recommended that in writing an historical case study, one should "adopt the following procedure: (1) one gives a rational reconstruction; (2) one tries to compare this rational reconstruction with actual history and to criticize both one's rational reconstruction for lack of historicity and the actual history for lack of rationality" (Lakatos, 1968, p. 138).

My goal is to provide a rational reconstruction, in what I take to be the Lakatosian sense, of what has aptly been described as "a vast historical catastrophe, the collapse of ancient medicine" (Wootton, 2007, p. 13). My reconstruction is based entirely on what contemporary physicians *wrote*, that is, it is based on the analysis of texts. In this sense, my project is strictly *philosophical*. However, I am perfectly willing to acknowledge that other reconstructions of these events may be possible. So, in a sense, my account can also be seen as a collection of historical hypotheses, and, as any hypotheses, mine can be tested empirically. Thus, my account can be evaluated and challenged both historically and philosophically. But whether my account proves to be adequate on either ground, it is, at the very least, one way of making some sense of an absolutely crucial episode in the history of medical science, an episode that has received far too little attention from either historians or philosophers.

Here is the course my account will take: the first two chapters will describe and explain the role of therapeutic bloodletting in early nineteenth-century medicine. Since bloodletting was conceived of both as a prophylaxis and as a therapy, this investigation will lead us, in chapter 3, directly to the nineteenth-century concepts of disease and disease causation. By that point, it will be clear that traditional medicine, including bloodletting, was mostly a system for reinforcing social and moral norms. This means, of course, that the effectiveness of traditional medicine cannot be adequately appraised simply in terms of what we would now regard as therapeutic success. In chapter 4, this interpretation of traditional medicine will receive some ancillary support from what may seem to be a rather unlikely source: the early nineteenth-century concept of quackery. Everywhere and always, regular practitioners have distinguished themselves from quacks, but the basis for the distinction has not always been the same. Historians have acknowledged that earlier conceptions of quackery must have been different from our own, although few seem to have grasped exactly what the differences were. Once it is clear how quacks were conceived of in the early nineteenth century, it will be apparent that, at that time, what we would now classify as therapeutic success had little to do with the effectiveness of medicine and that medicine was primarily a matter of reinforcing norms. Chapter 5 concerns a crucial historical episode known as the Edinburgh bloodletting controversy. This controversy began in the early 1850s. Among the issues that were prominent in the ensuing debate was the reason for the decline of therapeutic bloodletting, a decline that was already well underway by the time the controversy began. We will see that most of the physicians who participated in this controversy ascribed the decline of bloodletting to a change in their clientele—a change in the patients whom they were called upon to treat. This change, which can be traced to contemporary social and economic developments, dramatically reduced the number of cases in which bloodletting seemed to be the appropriate therapy. Chapter 6 concerns a change in how diseases were conceived; this semantic change can be dated to the early 1830s, although its most prominent and influential examples appeared near the middle of the century. In Chapter 7, we will see how this conceptual change ultimately proved to be the final blow in the demise of the traditional therapies and of Hippocratic medicine in general. At that point, it will be clear why the collapse of traditional medicine was a true precondition for the rise of the germ theory of disease and of scientific medicine. Finally, in Chapter 8, we will encounter some criticisms of our current way of conceiving disease and consider what the possible outcomes of these criticisms may be.

1

Bloodletting and Inflammation

Bloodletting, "the single greatest error in the history of medicine," was abandoned only after "the claim that it is beneficial was tested and refuted."
—Joseph Agassi (1969)

Whatever explanation may be given of the effects of bloodletting, there is no doubt of its multiplied results in the treatment of disease.
—James Wardrop (1833)

At 9:00 p.m. on July 13, 1824, a twenty-one-year-old sergeant in a French regiment of infantry was stabbed through the chest while engaged in single combat. His right carotid artery was punctured, and within minutes, he was unconscious from loss of blood. The bleeding was controlled by "very forcible compression," and the sergeant was quickly transported to a local hospital. At half past nine, "the patient was placed in bed, his head and shoulders being raised by pillows. He was immediately bled from the arm to 20 ounces." At one o'clock in the morning, "a second bleeding was ordered to the amount of twelve ounces," and two hours later, another twelve ounces were taken. The chief physician, Professor Jacques Mathieu Delpech, arrived at seven in the morning; he ordered an immediate bleeding of ten ounces and five more bleedings of eight or ten ounces each followed at regular intervals through the next fourteen hours. Altogether, in the first twenty-four hours after admission, in addition to the blood lost on the field of battle, his medical attendants systematically removed ninety ounces of the sergeant's blood. The specific gravity of blood is 1.060, so sixteen ounces of blood are almost one pint. Thus, in the first day of treatment, more than half the sergeant's normal supply of blood (about ten pints) was deliberately drained away. Two days later, on July 16, eighteen more ounces were taken; on each of the next

9

two days, he was bled a further eight ounces and on July 24, another twelve ounces. The wound remained sore and swollen, and by July 29, it was evident to Delpech that "suppurative inflammation had commenced." He ordered twelve leeches applied to the most sensitive part of the wound, and, later in the day, twenty more leeches were applied to the same area. The next afternoon, "four ounces of blood escaped [from the wound] in a large jet"; in response to this accident, four more ounces were drained and more leeches were applied. Over the next three days, a total of forty more leeches were applied to the most painful part of the wound. "Towards the end of September, the strength of the patient had very much returned; he left his bed and could take a little exercise." He was discharged from the hospital on October 3. Delpech concluded that "by the large quantity of blood lost, amounting to 170 ounces [nearly eleven pints], besides that drawn by the application of [a total of seventy-two] leeches [perhaps another two pints], the life of the patient was preserved." By contemporary standards, two hundred ounces of blood taken over the space of a few months was a large but by no means exceptional quantity of blood; the medical literature of the period contains many similar accounts—some successful, some not. Delpech found this case novel enough to warrant publication, not because of the massive bleedings, but because digitalis had been used as a sedative "in much larger doses than have ever been tried in this country" (Delpech, 1825). How are we to understand such medical treatment? What could the medical attendants possibly have been thinking?

Bloodletting can be explained on at least two levels. In this chapter, we will consider the practice in relation to what were called inflammatory symptoms; this explanation, while relatively superficial, will be sufficient to answer some basic questions about how bloodletting was used and why it was deemed to be effective. In chapter 2, we will examine the practice in a broader context and present a more comprehensive justification of its use.

I

As is illustrated in the account of the infantry sergeant's treatment, bloodletting occurred in two forms: sometimes, using a special instrument called a lancet, physicians opened a vein or an artery and simply allowed the patient's blood to flow into a receptacle. This approach, which was called venesection, phlebotomy, or general bloodletting, was usually selected when a patient was feverish or was judged to be at risk to become so. The sergeant in the previous account was repeatedly bled in this way presumably to prevent the onset of fever. In other cases, those in which a patient had a local inflammation on the surface of the body, physicians removed blood directly from the inflamed tissues. This was called local bloodletting, and it could be done either by abrading the skin and applying suction in one way or another or by applying leeches to the inflamed tissues. In the sergeant's case, when his wound became inflamed, leeches were applied directly to the surface of the wound.

Bloodletting, local, general, or a combination of both, was central to a broader therapeutic strategy called the antiphlogistic regimen. The name comes from the word *phlogiston* which, in a now antiquated and discarded theory of physics, referred to the hypothetical essence of fire, heat, or inflammability. When nineteenth-century physicians observed fever or inflamed tissues, it seemed reasonable to suppose that the patient was generally or locally overheated; the antiphlogistic regimen was conceived of as removing excess heat, and a central part of the process was removing blood. Beyond bloodletting, the regimen could also include such measures as purging, blistering, dietary restrictions, and the use of cooling lotions. Since a large number of medical problems involved fever or inflammation, the antiphlogistic regimen and bloodletting in particular were central to much of medical practice.

One four-volume medical encyclopedia, which included articles by fifty of England's most celebrated physicians and which went through several editions beginning in 1830, recommended the antiphlogistic regimen, and bloodletting in particular, for about two-thirds of the diseases identified in the index. These included acne, apoplexy (now called stroke), asthma, beriberi, cancer, cholera, chorea, coma, convulsions, croup, diabetes, difficult teething, dropsy, dysentery, eczema, emphysema, epilepsy, gangrene, gout, hemorrhoids, hepatitis, herpes, hiccup, hydrophobia (now called rabies), indigestion, insanity, jaundice, laryngitis, leprosy, ophthalmia, palpitations of the heart, paralysis, phthisis (now called tuberculosis), plague, pleurisy, pneumonia, rheumatism, scurvy, smallpox, softening of the brain, spinal meningitis, suppression of urine, tetanus, tonsillitis, and whooping cough, as well as eleven different forms of hemorrhage and about seventy other assorted disorders (Forbes, Tweedie, and Conolly, 1849). "Even during surgical operations, doctors viewed bleeding (artificial or hemorrhaging) as beneficial in preventing febrile symptoms and local inflammation . . .. Before amputations it was common to bleed patients to the extent that the loss of blood would equal the amount estimated to circulate in the limb" (Haller, 1982, p. 49). And, of course, there is the revealing fact that the medical journal *Lancet*, which was founded in 1823 and which remains one of the world's most prominent medical journals, was named after the instrument by which venesection was performed.

How extensive was therapeutic bloodletting in the early decades of the century? In 1859, one American physician estimated that, over the course of his career, he had removed more than one hundred barrels of blood (Haller, 1982, p. 49). The number of leeches in use also gives some indication of the extent of bloodletting: during this period, in addition to all the leeches that could be produced and harvested domestically (and the harvesting was so thorough that some physicians feared that leeches might actually become extinct), British physicians imported more than seven million leeches each year from such countries as France, Germany, Silesia, and Poland, and even from Turkey, Egypt, India, and Australia (Carter, 2001). (For purposes of comparison, in the 1830s, the population of Great Britain was about ten million.)

General bloodletting or venesection was relatively straightforward. It was simply a matter of opening a vein or an artery and allowing blood to flow. Of course, there were some risks. For one thing, there was always the danger of taking too much blood. This problem was generally controlled by bleeding patients while they were sitting erect in bed or even standing—the thinking was that as long as a patient could sit or stand erect, he or she had not yet lost so much blood as to be in danger; once the patient passed out, it was time to stop. However, it was widely recognized that, by accident, patients were sometimes literally bled to death. This was suspected to have happened, for example, both to George Washington and to his contemporary, King George III of England. Another related problem was that it was sometimes difficult to stop the flow of blood once it had begun. Practitioners were cautioned to be prepared to arrest the flow of blood by stitching the opening together with a needle and silk thread or by employing cauterizing agents, ligatures, or plaster of Paris.

Local bloodletting was a more complex procedure and one whose success depended on the mastery of some rather specialized techniques—techniques that were continually being scrutinized and perfected in the early decades of the nineteenth century. One way of bleeding locally was by abrading the skin to expose inflamed tissues and by applying mechanical devices that created enough suction to withdraw blood. However, the most effective and most popular means of bleeding locally was by the application of leeches. When brought into contact with a living animal, a leech punctures its victim's skin with a bite that resembles the emblem on a Mercedes-Benz. It then secretes various anesthetic, anticoagulant, and diffusing agents, and for about half an hour, it sucks the blood that flows from its host. Tests conducted in the early nineteenth century indicated that a leech would consume about half an ounce of blood before detaching itself. However, the use of leeches was not as simple as one might expect. In 1804, G. Wilkinson recommended that the area to which leeches were to be applied should be washed with soap and water, rinsed thoroughly, and, when appropriate, shaved very close to the skin: "I have found the sharp points of the incised hairs so greatly to annoy them, as to prevent their fixing." He observed that leeches could best be controlled by placing them in a wine glass; this was useful not only "for observing their motions, circumscribing their limits, retaining them in the proper place assigned for their bite, but it also tends to support them when filling and thereby prevents their separating from the parts sooner than they otherwise would do." If leeches were reluctant to bite, they could be encouraged by rubbing the target area with sugar water, milk, or, most effective of all, a small quantity of fresh blood. A few years later, one practitioner reported that submerging leeches in diluted wine or, very briefly, in warm full-strength porter would cause them to bite and suck vigorously (Wilkinson, 1848). If a leech became attached at the wrong site (or "what is equally bad" on the practitioner's fingers), it could be made to release its hold by sprinkling table salt on its mouth.

Leeches were deemed especially useful in removing blood from areas of the body that were too constricted to allow for the application of mechanical suction—areas such as in and around the nose and ears, inside the mouth, and within the rectum and vagina. They were sometimes also used to achieve the benefits of general bloodletting in infants or in patients who were too weak to withstand venesection. When substituting for general bleeding, the usual procedure was to place one or more leeches as near as possible to the focus of the morbid process: for headache, on the temples; for gastrointestinal inflammation, on the abdomen; for bladder troubles, on the shaved pubis; and for menstrual disorders, on the thighs, the groin, and the vulva.

Through the early nineteenth century, there was considerable interest in improving techniques for removing blood from different parts of the body. William Brown observed that while morbid accumulations of blood in the head or in the lower belly were often relieved, by nature, through repeated spontaneous bleeding from the nose or from the rectum, physicians needed to develop alternative methods for use when these "efforts of nature" were inadequate. He recommended the following procedure for taking blood from the hemorrhoidal veins—a procedure he described as well-established in many parts of Europe. The patient

> is seated on a perforated chair, which only uncovers the anus itself; the operator, stooping or kneeling, by means of a taper, sees the part to which the leech is to be applied; and, provided with a small round wide-bottomed bottle with a long neck, just large enough to contain one leech, he allows the animal to draw out and fix itself on the part intended. The operator having applied one leech, withdraws the bottle, and proceeds to fix one after another till the desired number have been applied; a basin is placed under the chair into which the blood flows (Brown, 1818, p. 140).

Brown pointed out that this technique was useful in most abdominal inflammations "such as hepatitis, enteritis, [and] puerperal fever, [as well as] in suppressed menses, lochia, etc."

Since the mucous membranes often became inflamed, it seemed desirable to apply leeches to these tissues as well. Philip Crampton reported applying leeches directly to inflamed tonsils, but this procedure involved obvious risks: for one thing, the leeches could become detached and accidentally suffocate the patient. He explained that to avoid such an accident, he passed a single thread of silk

> through the body of the leech, at about its lower third, the ligature being made fast to the finger of the operator, the leech . . . was introduced into the mouth, and its head, directed by a probe, was brought into contact with the inflamed tonsil. The animal fixed itself to the part in an instant, and, in less than five minutes, being gorged with blood, it fell upon the tongue, and was withdrawn (Crampton, 1822, p. 229).

A later physician reported that passing threads through leeches, "far from incapacitating them from action, causes them to bite with increased ardor, and, in fact, [the procedure] may be used to stimulate torpid leeches." Crampton reported that when leeches were applied directly to the tonsils, "relief [to the patient] was immediate." He also found that the application of leeches to the internal surface of the nostrils provided the greatest possible relief in cases of "undue determination of blood to the brain" or in cases of habitual nosebleed.

A decade later, in 1833, John Osborne praised Crampton's pioneering work and recommended several improvements of his own. In bronchitis, he observed, "the application of leeches to the larynx and to the trachea in the triangular space between the mastoid muscles, has appeared . . . to be the most decisive and immediately successful remedy of all those I have ever applied." This use of leeches was also effective in laryngitis and was "of singular efficacy in stopping the cough of phthisis [a disorder now classified as a form of tuberculosis], in so much that by resorting to it . . . we have enabled to secure sleep at night, and during the day to keep the phthisical patients so free from cough that a superficial observer might readily believe that we had cured the disease." Osborn also noted that leeches would continue to suck when submerged in water "at a temperature considerably above 100 degrees." This meant that a patient could be placed in a warm bath for treatment; when the leeches finished sucking and dropped off, the warm water ensured that the bites continued to bleed so that even more blood was extracted.

Osborn felt that his own most valuable contribution to leechcraft was in solving a problem that had long vexed physicians: "In treating intestinal inflammation, the application of leeches to the anus had little effect, and to apply them internally is often difficult, on account of the violent contractions of the sphincter." Osborne overcame this difficulty by the use of a grooved metal rod (with an elegant leather handle), which he designed and ordered to be constructed especially for the purpose. In using the rod, Osborn explained, one first passed a thread through the tail of the leech (as Crampton had recommended a decade earlier). The leech was then placed in the groove of the instrument and,

> the operator, holding the ends of the threads, introduces the instrument into the rectum, and pushes it up so as to cause it to draw up the leeches along with it into the rectum. When they have thus been conveyed up beyond the sphincter, the instrument is withdrawn, and the leeches are suffered to remain till gorged with blood and loosened from their hold, when they are drawn out by means of the threads which the operator retains outside the anus. (Osborne, 1833, p. 339f)

Osborne observed, "I have never used more than four leeches at once, in this way, fearing lest too great a hemorrhage might be produced." He noted that such devices also allowed leeches to be applied directly to enlarged prostate glands.

Leeches were regularly introduced into the vagina to stimulate menstrual flow and to treat various feminine disorders. One obstetrician, Samuel Ashwell, observed that leeches applied directly "to the *os uteri* . . . [were] decidedly more beneficial than any other local depletion" (Ashwell, 1852). He pointed out that "the speculum tube may be introduced into the vagina prior to their application; and if the cervix be brought fully into view, neither the vagina nor any other part than this portion of the congested viscus will be fixed on by the leeches." Ashwell recommended that this indelicate use of leeches be "confined to married women" and that "a clever nurse should be taught to apply them."

Treating a single disease episode usually required only a few leeches; however, sometimes many more seemed to be indicated. "A gentleman [who] fell from his horse and severely bruised the elbow-joint" was treated by the application of 118 leeches over the course of four days (Wardrop, 1833–4). Between July 22 and August 3, 1824, 130 leeches were applied to the inflamed testicles of a patient with gonorrhea (Tyrrell, 1824). In four days, 160 leeches were applied to the abdomen of one woman in an unsuccessful attempt to save her from puerperal fever (Editor's Note, 1828–9); however, one year earlier, a case of severe metritis "was subdued by the application of 220 leeches and two venesections within ten days" (White, 1819).

Various difficulties and risks were associated with the use of leeches. Leech bites, an obvious indication of recent medical treatment, could be embarrassing. Referring to treatment of testicular inflammation, Astley Cooper, a prominent surgeon, observed that in private practice, he saw "persons in whom it is of the greatest consequence that a bleeding from these parts should be concealed" (Cooper, 1823–4). Cooper recommended that in treating such persons, rather than leeching, one should use a lancet to carefully open a few veins in the scrotum. As in general bleeding, leeching also sometimes led to the removal of too much blood. One physician, "desirous of being enabled to get about among [his] patients as speedily as possible, applied sixty leeches to his own sprained ankle which he then soaked in hot water." "The consequence," he reported, "was not merely a faintness, like death, from which no measures could for half an hour or more restore me, but an excessive degree of general debility, from which I did not recover entirely for months" (Grower, 1831–2).

An equally serious hazard was that leeches applied to the throat could suffocate patients, or be swallowed and then attach themselves within the lower esophagus, "thereby causing extensive mischief" (Editor's Review, 1842–3). Another problem was that leech bites sometimes bled so profusely as to become life-threatening. Anthony White reported that a two-year-old girl had died from the loss of blood induced by a single leech (White, 1819), and similar deaths were occasionally reported throughout the early decades of the century. Physicians recommended that, where possible, leeches should be applied over solid internal tissue, such as a bone, so that pressure could be applied to stop the bleeding. Physicians were also cautioned to be prepared to stop the flow of blood by the same methods that could be used if too much blood was released in venesection.

Another risk was that the leech bite could itself become the focus of subsequent morbid processes. One physician advised against applying leeches to the eyelids, or to the scrotum or penis, because he had seen "very violent inflammation, and even gangrene, result from it, . . . an accident by which the reputation of the surgeon cannot fail to suffer" (Lisfranc, 1836). He also observed that leech bites could give rise to erysipelas and other inflammatory processes. In another essay, the same physician argued against the use of leeches in uterine disorders since they were seldom beneficial and the bites "easily changed into as many cancerous ulcerations" (Lisfranc, 1833–4). There was also a persisting concern that reused leeches could themselves convey diseases from one person to another. Early in the century, Wilkinson discounted the notion that leeches, "which may have been previously applied to patients in the small-pox, measles, scarlet fever, venereal buboes, or other affections of this sort, or to cancerous, venereal, or phagedenic ulcers, bites of a mad dog, or any other specific disease whatever, will or can communicate a similar affection" (Wilkinson, 1848). However, publications occasionally suggested otherwise: one editorial reported that leeches had conveyed syphilis to a child after being used to treat a syphilitic patient (Editor's Note, 1827–8).

II

So how, if at all, could bloodletting have been justified? In answering this question, we are not interested in explaining away the special risks or potential abuses of bloodletting (as illustrated in the preceding three paragraphs): after all, some risk and the possibility of abuse are inherent in any medical intervention, justified or not. Rather, our concern is with therapeutic bloodletting as a general practice.

Of course, many modern critics have rejected bloodletting as entirely unwarranted. Joseph Agassi denounced bloodletting as "the single greatest error in the history of medicine" and held that the practice was abandoned only after "the claim that bleeding is beneficial was tested and refuted" (Agassi, 1969, p. 159). As will become apparent, both assertions are false. David Wootton adopted a more nuanced position. He acknowledged that bloodletting probably had some value as a placebo. Since doctors and their patients believed in the practice, by "mobilizing the body's own resources" it may in some cases have actually promoted healing (Wootton, 2007, p. 68). Of course, even with this concession, Wootton still does not believe that bloodletting was justified; he explains that

> bloodletting, purging, and emetics acted powerfully and, in so far as they acted on the body, they were bad for patients, but we can be confident that if one tested Hippocratic remedies against placebos the placebos would outperform the Hippocratic remedies: doing worse than a placebo is, if you like, a technical definition of what I am calling "bad medicine" or "doing harm." By this definition, . . . you are doing harm even if your patient is more likely to recover as a result of receiving your treatment than if he had received no treatment at all, providing your treatment is less beneficial than a placebo (Wootton, 2007, p. 68).

Near the end of his book, Wootton elaborates his conclusion that bloodletting was bad medicine: "If we define medicine as the ability to cure diseases, then there was very little medicine before 1865. The long tradition that descended from Hippocrates, symbolized by a reliance on bloodletting, purges, and emetics, was almost totally ineffectual, indeed positively deleterious, except in so far as it mobilized the placebo effect" (Wootton, 2007, p. 283).

In the preceding quotation, Wootton acknowledges that his conclusion—namely the conclusion that (except for a possible placebo effect) bloodletting was ineffective or even harmful—depends on the assumption that, throughout history, medicine can be understood as the ability to cure disease. At first glance, this assumption seems reasonable—what else could medicine be about? But sometimes the most plausible assumptions turn out to be false or at least misleading. According to this assumption, physicians throughout history have all shared the same one objective—the only difference is that, while we are now somewhat successful, for two thousand years, practitioners just plain got it wrong and actually did their patients harm. But surely the idea of a two-thousand-year quest that consistently did more harm than good seems a bit . . . implausible. Must one not begin to wonder whether earlier medical practice, and in particular bloodletting, was actually achieving something other than what we now think of as curing disease? If so, then even if bloodletting was ineffective in this one sense, it might have achieved other worthwhile benefits—benefits that do not fall under this heading. In this case, simply dismissing bloodletting as bad medicine (even if true, given suitable definitions and assumptions) would provide only a distorted picture of what was actually happening. Indeed, could an earlier physician not make the argument that our system of medicine is ineffective or harmful since it does not achieve whatever goals the earlier physicians may have sought?

Moreover, Wootton's argument surely depends on a second assumption as well, namely, on the assumption that the word *disease* must be taken in the sense in which we now understand it. What if bloodletting actually did cure disease, but only if we take the word *disease* to mean something subtly different from what the word now means? If so, then even if we grant the first assumption (the assumption that bloodletting was intended to cure disease), and even if, from our point of view, bloodletting was bad medicine, the practice may actually have been effective against diseases as they were formerly conceived; indeed, it may have worked extremely well. In this case, once again, simply dismissing bloodletting as bad medicine on the grounds that it fails to cure what we now call disease would be seriously misleading. In short, in rejecting bloodletting as bad medicine, one is assuming both that bloodletting was intended to cure disease and that diseases were conceived very much as we now conceive them. These are reasonable assumptions, and one can certainly use the word *medicine* in this sense if one chooses to do so; what I maintain is that by making these assumptions, one seriously misrepresents bloodletting and the entire medical system of which it was a part. Given a more sympathetic understanding of the practice, it becomes clear that therapeutic bloodletting could have achieved much more than a mere placebo.

So how did early nineteenth-century physicians conceive of disease? Answering this question will enable us to decide how, if at all, bloodletting could have been effective against diseases as they were then understood. In chapter 2, we will consider whether early nineteenth-century medicine can fairly be appraised using the standards that we would now use to evaluate medical care—thus, in the second chapter, we will ask whether early nineteenth-century medicine was really about curing disease at all.

So how, in fact, were diseases conceived two hundred years ago? In the early nineteenth century, most diseases were regarded as nothing more than collections of disordered states of the body. "Disease is the disordered action of any part of the machinery of the body. Its primary effects, or perhaps we should say, its primary palpable phenomena, are impeded or disordered functions" (Conolly, 1849, p. 674). What does this mean? And how, if at all, does it differ from our current conception? We can best answer these questions by looking at a particular disease. Any number of examples can be found in every English, French, or German medical text published in the period. We will consider the discussion of one typical disease (ophthalmia) in one typical medical text (William Buchan's *Domestic Medicine or a Treatise on the Prevention and Cure of Disease*).

Buchan's *Domestic Medicine* was first published in 1769; by 1805, when Buchan died, the book had gone through nineteen English editions and sold about eighty thousand copies (roughly one for every one hundred persons then living in Great Britain); the book was translated into all the main European languages, and it was praised by the medical community as well as by distinguished laypersons. Catherine the Great, Empress of Russia, awarded Buchan a gold medal in recognition of the humanitarian value of the publication (Dunn, 2000). At his death, Buchan was buried in Westminster Abbey—an honor reserved for England's greatest heroes. The book certainly represents a fair sample of common medical opinion, lay and professional, at the beginning of the nineteenth century.

Buchan defines *ophthalmia* as inflammation of the eye, and *inflammation* meant, as it does for us today, redness, heat, swelling, and pain, in this case, of the eye (Buchan, 1779, p. 282). Near the beginning of his discussion, Buchan explains that ophthalmia "may be occasioned by external injuries; as strokes, dust, quicklime, or the like, thrown into the eyes. . . . too long exposure to the night air, especially in cold northerly winds, or whatever suddenly checks perspiration . . . [by] viewing snow or other white bodies for a long time, or looking steadfastly at the sun, a clear fire, or any bright object. . . . [by] drinking spirituous liquors and excess of venery . . . [or by] the acrid fumes of metals, and of several kinds of fuel . . . [It] sometimes . . . proceeds from a venereal taint, and often from a scrofulous or gouty habit. It may likewise be occasioned by hairs in the eye-lids turning inwards, and hurting the eyes. Sometimes the disease is epidemic, especially after wet seasons; and I have frequently known it to prove infectious" (Buchan, 1779, p. 281f).

We, today, would see a wide range of different and largely unrelated problems here—in our terms, Buchan seems to be lumping together as one disorder, various physical and chemical irritations, reactions to intoxication, numerous possible infections, probably even some hereditary issues; yet in each case, Buchan sees only ophthalmia—inflammation of the eye. We, today, are accustomed to distinguishing between physical ailments based largely on their underlying causes; Buchan lists numerous diverse possible causes of ophthalmia, but then, in respect to diagnosis and treatment, he altogether ignores the causes and focuses exclusively on the common "disordered state," in this case, on redness, heat, swelling, and pain in the eye. To make sense of bloodletting, it is essential to think of disease as Buchan did—as a particular disordered state of the body and nothing more. If ophthalmia is only this disordered state, that is, the inflammatory symptoms, any treatment that removes these symptoms is an effective treatment for the disease. In cases of ophthalmia, irrespective of its causes, whatever removes inflammation of the eye effectively cures the disease.

In our terms, today, local inflammation—which is still defined as redness, heat, swelling, and pain—is said to occur when, from whatever underlying cause, the arterioles in a specific area contract, the associated capillaries dilate and become flushed with blood, and blood, including plasma proteins and leukocytes, passes into the surrounding tissues. One way of reducing local inflammation is by removing this excess blood and its associated fluids—removing blood reverses inflammation by reducing redness, heat, and swelling, and, to some extent, it may also reduce pain. This is a fact. Indeed, it comes close to being true by definition, and it has never been disputed—it is as true now as it was in Buchan's day. Even today, one means of reducing local inflammation is by removing blood and other fluids from the inflamed area (although we usually prefer other therapies such as ice packs or anti-inflammatory drugs such as ibuprofen). In Buchan's day, to say that bloodletting was effective against local inflammation *meant* that it was effective against diseases like ophthalmia since diseases were merely the disordered state that comprised the symptoms. In our

21

day, insofar as inflammatory symptoms are themselves regarded as a morbid process, it is still effective against that form of morbidity; however, if we think of disease as something other than the symptoms (e.g., as an underlying infection), bloodletting may seem to provide, as best, a modest and temporary benefit. So, depending on the results we are trying to achieve—depending on how we define *disease*—local bloodletting may or may not be truly effective.

A similar argument can be made concerning fever, the usual target of general bloodletting. As nineteenth-century physicians explained it, venesection seemed to reduce fever by first "producing a diminution of nervous power . . . second . . . by lessening the quantity of blood. . . . [and] third . . . by facilitating the reestablishment of the secreting functions" (Cooper, 1823). We, today, recognize that a patient who loses a significant amount of blood experiences what is sometimes called "peripheral shut down"—blood is retained within the central organs, the extremities become cool and may even begin to turn blue. This produces a definite and perceptible cooling effect. Once again, if one is concerned only to reduce fever, one way of doing it is by abstracting blood. It is an indisputable fact, today, as it was two hundred years ago, that removing a significant amount of blood will generally lower the body temperature of a patient. Once again, if fever itself (as opposed to some underlying problem like a bacterial infection) is seen as the ultimate target of treatment—as, indeed, it was seen in early nineteenth-century medicine—then general bloodletting is truly effective. In this respect, there is no doubt that, from their point of view, earlier physicians were correct.

Nineteenth-century physicians were certain that local and general bloodletting worked. It was described as "the most powerful means of relieving inflammation" (Cooper, 1823). And their confidence was based on experience, not on theoretical arguments—they believed in bloodletting because they saw that it worked (Clutterbuck, 1826, p. 7). For this reason, the fact that the effectiveness of bloodletting could not be fully explained was not seen as a problem. One physician referred to "the wild and untenable" (later "wild and baseless") theories by which "innumerable theorists of every kind, as well as . . . those who were no theorists at all" tried to explain the effectiveness of bleeding, and was "quite willing . . . to make a bonfire of all that has been written for and against bloodletting from a theoretical point of view" (Gairdner, 1857–8, pp. 206f, 208). But physicians agreed that "whatever explanation may be given of the effects of bloodletting, there is no doubt of its multiplied results in the treatment of disease" (Wardrop, 1833, p. 237). Ironically, the absence of agreement as to how bloodletting achieved its benefits was, itself, seen as a kind of confirmation of its effectiveness: "If three men are all equally sure of the efficacy of a remedy, and each of the three has an entirely different hypothesis as to its action, the probability is, that there is some basis in experience for the *fact* which they all profess to hold as true, notwithstanding the diversity of their theoretical interpretation" (Gairdner, 1857–8, p. 207).

Thus, while Buchan would have been unable to explain the mechanism of inflammation in the terms we would use today, he understood quite clearly, and confirmed repeatedly in his everyday practice, that removing blood reduced inflammation. So, logically enough, for cases of ophthalmia, Buchan recommended a combination of general and local bloodletting: "Bleeding, in a violent inflammation of the eyes, is always necessary. This should be performed as near to the part affected as possible. An adult may lose ten or twelve ounces of blood from the jugular vein" (Buchan, 1779, p. 283). Today, one might object that even if such a treatment helped, any benefit could be only temporary; surely, unless the underlying cause was corrected, inflammation would immediately return once the bloodletting ceased. Buchan understood perfectly well that inflammation frequently returned after treatment and so the previous quotation continues, "and the operation [i.e., bloodletting] may be repeated according to the urgency of the symptoms." In other words, as inflammation returns, take more blood, and, by implication, continue doing so until the inflammation ceases (just as, today, a patient may be instructed to apply ice packs to a swollen ankle and to continue the treatment until the swelling subsides). "If it should not be convenient to bleed in the neck, the same quantity may be let from the arm, or any other part of the body. Leeches are often applied to the temples, or under the eyes, with good effect. The wounds must be suffered to bleed for some hours, and if the bleeding stops soon, it may be promoted by the application of cloths dipped in warm water. In obstinate cases, it will be necessary to repeat this operation several times" (Buchan, 1779, p. 284).

So on one level, justifying bloodletting is as simple as that: the disordered state that Buchan called ophthalmia is a kind of inflammation, bloodletting reverses inflammation, therefore, bloodletting is an effective treatment for ophthalmia. No one who understands these words (at least no one who understands the words in the sense in which Buchan did) could doubt this conclusion. However temporary, bloodletting was an effective treatment for ophthalmia. Since many diseases involved inflammatory symptoms, similar reasoning implied that bloodletting was very widely applicable.

By 1822, medical professionals had improved on the treatment Buchan recommended. Philip Crampton, "surgeon in ordinary to the King, surgeon general to the army and forces in Ireland, etc.," acknowledged that local bloodletting is "among the most effective means which art supplies for the relief of local inflammation" (Crampton, 1822, p. 223), and he sought to improve the technique of local bloodletting. Based on a study of ophthalmic patients in the Royal Military Infirmary, Dublin, between 1814 and 1821, Crampton reported that "in a large majority of these cases (which included every kind and degree of inflammation of the eye) leeches were repeatedly applied to the conjunctiva [!] . . . and I can distinctly state, that not only in no instance was the practice attended with any inconvenience, but that in by far the greatest number of cases, the application of one, or at the utmost two leeches to the conjunctiva, had a more decisive effect in unloading the inflamed and turgid vessels of that membrane, than the application of five times that number to the temple and eyelids" (Crampton, 1822, p. 227). Crampton also reported favorable results— success, as he put it, beyond his "most sanguine expectations"—from applying leeches to the external fauces (tissues between the soft palate and the base of the tongue) in the case of sore throat, or directly to the inflamed tonsils in the case of tonsillitis. No one who understands Crampton's claims can doubt that they are true. Moreover, in comparison to Buchan's recommendations, Crampton's therapies mark true medical progress—indeed, in a sense, *evidence-based progress*: Crampton identified treatments that were more effective than those recommended by Buchan, and he had confirmed this in numerous (randomly selected?) patients over many years. Bloodletting was definitely better than a placebo.

So was the application of leeches really beneficial? Was it good or bad medicine? The answer is not a simple matter of fact. A lot depends on how we conceive of disease. Even if we adopt a modern point of view, bloodletting may well reduce inflammation more effectively than a placebo (although so far as I know neither this nor the opposite conclusion has ever been confirmed empirically). However, if we adopt Buchan's point of view, the answer is indisputable. For Buchan, the disease was exactly the disordered state of the body, so whatever corrects this disordered state is an effective treatment. For Buchan, any therapy that diminishes the disorder must qualify as good medicine, and bloodletting indubitably does so. End of story.

III

By now it should be obvious that it is not a simple matter to show that bloodletting was ineffective. Indeed, if we adopt the assumptions of early nineteenth-century medicine, such a demonstration would probably be impossible. This is because, from the earlier point of view, as a treatment for inflammation (as a treatment for the specific physical disorder that it was intended to treat), bloodletting clearly worked. However, this reasoning does not entail that absolutely no nineteenth-century arguments could have been used against bloodletting. For example, even then one could have argued that bloodletting did not reduce the duration or the severity of symptoms—perhaps patients would have recovered from ophthalmia just as quickly or even more quickly without bloodletting. One could also argue that, since our modern point of view is, after all, correct or at least better than the early nineteenth-century way of thinking, the fact that earlier physicians could not argue against bloodletting simply illustrates the inadequacy of their medical system—perhaps they didn't understand that diseases are different from sets of symptoms, but they *should* have. We will return to this second kind of argument in chapter 2. For now we will consider only the possibility of arguments of the first kind: Could someone have argued against (or possibly for) bloodletting by determining whether bloodletting affected the duration or the severity of symptoms?

In fact, in 1828, one French clinical epidemiologist, Pierre-Charles-Alexandre Louis, reported just such a study. In that year, Louis published a paper entitled "Research on the effects of bloodletting in some inflammatory diseases" (Louis, 1828). Seven years later, in 1835, a slightly revised and expanded version of the paper appeared as a book; in 1836, the book was translated into English. At present, one occasionally encounters the opinion that Louis's publications were a serious challenge, indeed, the first scientific challenge, to bloodletting. At least at the time of this writing, this is the view presented on Wikipedia, and it can also be found in more serious histories (Ackerknecht, 1946, p. 134). But the facts do not warrant this opinion.

In his publications, Louis considered three inflammatory diseases: pneumonia, erysipelas of the face, and angina tonsillaris. His results are similar for each disease, and we will focus on his remarks about pneumonia. Louis reported having examined seventy-seven cases in which pneumonia had been treated by bloodletting; he divided these cases into patients who had been bled within the first four days of the onset of symptoms and those whose treatment had commenced only later. He found that patients who were treated early on, recovered, on average, three days sooner than those not bled until later. This result, far from discrediting bloodletting, actually supports its use—at least if blood is taken in a timely manner. However, Louis's study also revealed something else, something that he, personally, found "startling and apparently absurd": of those who were bled early, 44 percent died, while of the patients whose treatment had commenced later, only 25 percent died. Louis was unsure what to make of this result, but he acknowledged two factors that may have influenced the finding: first, by chance, the patients who had been bled early happened, on average, to be significantly older (and so may have been weaker and more vulnerable to death) than those who were bled late. Second, it was possible that those who were bled late may already have survived the most dangerous part of the illness and so may have been in the process of recovery when treatment commenced. This would mean that, on average, they would have had a more favorable prognosis than those bled earlier. Either of these factors could have explained the "startling and apparently absurd" result that patients bled early on died more frequently than those bled later. Yet, however this result was to be explained, Louis concluded, "the mortality and variations in the mean duration of pneumonia, based on the time at which bloodletting commenced, suggest that there are narrow limits to the effectiveness of this mode of treatment" (Louis, 1828, p. 323). In simple terms, Louis concluded that, to be effective, blood must be taken at just the proper time. But he himself did not infer that bloodletting was inappropriate; quite the contrary. He stressed that "both because of its influence on the state of the diseased organ, and because, in shortening the duration of the disease, it diminishes the chance of secondary lesions, it should not be neglected in inflammations that are severe and are seated in an important organ." He also commented that "the use of the lancet [i.e., general bleeding] should be preferred to that of leeches."

Louis's cautious and tentative conclusions hardly appear to be a significant challenge to the ancient and respected practice of bloodletting; indeed, current opinions notwithstanding, his results seem to support bloodletting rather than discrediting the practice, and that seems to be how he himself interpreted his findings. While Louis's argument is relatively weak (he had no real controls, his sample was far too small, and his cohorts seem to have been poorly chosen), his results actually provide some statistical support for the notion that bloodletting, when applied soon after the onset of symptoms, reduces the duration of the inflammatory diseases he considered. David Wootton observes that Louis's argument must, somehow, be wrong, "after all, if he was right, why do we not still let blood?" (Wootton, 2007, p. 173). It is difficult to decide how seriously to take this question. Does Wootton really mean that the realization that Louis's argument was defective, and that realization alone, led to the decline of bloodletting? Presumably not; such an interpretation makes no sense at all. Moreover, there is no reason to think that Louis's contemporaries found his argument defective. In any case, this underscores the striking absence of any significant argument against bloodletting in the literature of the early nineteenth century.

There is one more thing to say about the common contemporary opinion that Louis's arguments helped turn the tide of medical opinion against bloodletting. In chapter 5, we will review an episode known as the Edinburgh Bloodletting Controversy. This controversy resulted in scores of publications that appeared between 1850 and the end of the nineteenth century. The central purpose of most of these publications was to explain why bloodletting had declined precipitously—a decline that, by 1850, was taken already to be an established fact. Although Louis's book had been translated into English just a few years earlier, in 1836, and was known to the participants in the controversy, it was not taken as having provided conclusive evidence against the practice of bloodletting. So regardless of how Louis himself or his immediate contemporaries interpreted his results, it is far from clear that his publications had any significant impact on the decline of bloodletting.

And that's it. Beyond Louis's article and book, so far no document from the first half of the nineteenth century has been identified that challenges the general practice of bloodletting. Yet during those very decades, the practice was all but given up—given up by physicians who could not and did not doubt its effectiveness as a treatment for inflammation. Leon S. Bryan Jr. observes that the decline of bloodletting seems to have occurred without controversy or debate, that it was so subtle that many were unaware of the decline until after the practice had all but vanished, and that among those who did recognize what was happening, "no one seemed to know quite why" it was happening (Bryan, 1964). He notes that while isolated individuals argued against particular use of bloodletting (perhaps Bryan shared the common misinterpretation of Louis), their arguments were based on relatively little evidence and there is no reason to think that they significantly eroded confidence in the practice in general. Alex Berman observes, "One would like to regard the improvement in therapeutics [during the middle of the nineteenth century] as being part of a general scientific advance. The facts indicate, however, that scientific considerations played a minor role in demolishing the old heroic practice, and what was called 'rational' medication in 1860 was brought about largely by empirical and often irrational factors" (Berman, 1978, p. 79). Berman also quotes from contributors to a symposium conducted by the Philadelphia Country Medical Society in 1860 in which the reasons for the decline of bloodletting were discussed. One participant noted that the change took place

> involuntarily and unconsciously. No one can justify it . . . .. Not among any particular class of practitioners, nor among those of any particular country or place, but almost universally. The great body of the profession everywhere, and without previous interchange of views, we might almost say, without themselves being always aware of the fact, made bloodletting, to a certain extent, a subordinate remedy, even in diseases . . . in the treatment of which, but a short time before, it had been considered . . . the chief remedy. (Berman, 1978, p. 79)

So in bloodletting, we have a practice that was employed through centuries and that was then abandoned in the space of about one generation without anyone being able to justify or to explain why that happened. Not only that, it was abandoned by practitioners who did not and could not doubt that it was effective against inflammation— the very "disordered state" that it was intended to treat. How is this to be explained?

As I noted earlier, this entire chapter concerns only a relatively superficial interpretation of bloodletting. Even on this level of interpretation, it should now be apparent that the practice was not obviously or stupidly wrong—the practice was not simply a colossal mistake. But recognizing that bloodletting was more than a mistake makes it even more difficult to understand how it could have declined and vanished so suddenly and without any serious argument or debate. These are the main issues that this book is intended to address, but next, we must look at bloodletting from a different point of view, one that will reveal entirely different dimensions to the practice.

2

Bloodletting and Social Norms

The history of the treatment of hydrophobia [i.e., rabies], tetanus, epilepsy, etc. is a greater reflection on the art and science of medicine than the inability to cure.
—*Charles Simpson (1848)*

There ought to be some histories that show how the social order sustains itself, and how it sometimes does so without any of those who participate in the process fully understanding what they are doing.
—*David Wootton (2007)*

Blood: "a hot spark," "a man of fire," "a buck," a "fast or foppish man," "a rake." [The term appears] to arise from the sense [of blood as] the supposed seat of emotions, passions, but in many cases also associated with [blood in the sense of] blood worth mentioning, good blood, good parentage or stock [thus the term in this sense means] an aristocratic rowdy.
—*OED*

In her book, *Implicit Meanings*, Mary Douglas recounts an event that transpired while she was living among the Lele people of central Africa:

> In one case, an old widow was disputing the right to draw palm wine from a palm which had been planted by her late husband. The latter's sisters' sons ignored her claim, and started to draw the wine for themselves, arguing with her every time they met. One day one of the young men passing her hut on the way to draw the wine, was surprised to find her standing at the doorway, watching him in grim silence. He climbed the palm, and came down quickly in horror and disgust, reporting that he had put his hand into a mess of *tebe* [human excrement]. All the villagers were interested in the case; several climbed the palm to verify for themselves, and all agreed that it was indeed *tebe*, and that the palm would have to be abandoned.

The widow was accused of sorcery, and was eventually driven away from the village, a number of cases of recent deaths being laid to her charge. Her own kinsman, in her defense, asked how anyone supposed that a woman would be physical capable [sic] of climbing a tall palm and defecating on the top of it, but her enemies replied that the extraordinary feat was further proof of her mastery of the black arts of sorcery (Douglas, 1975, pp. 23–4).

Suppose one were to ask what was achieved by driving the old woman from the village? The Lele villagers themselves would likely answer that they had expelled a witch. By contrast, an outside observer might answer that, by labeling the woman a witch and driving her away, the villagers had ended a dispute that might otherwise have threatened the stability and coherence of their group—an achievement that could be of considerable benefit in a marginally viable society.

How does this apply to nineteenth-century medicine? Whether a medical practice like bloodletting is *beneficial* depends on the *benefits* that the practice actually yields, and it is entirely possible that, as in the case of expelling the Lele witch, a practice could benefit a society in ways quite different from those that the medical practitioners themselves might identify as their immediate goals. If asked, nineteenth-century practitioners—like physicians today—might very well have identified their goals as something like extending life or decreasing morbidity (perhaps by controlling inflammation). But in deciding whether nineteenth-century medical practice, including bloodletting, was beneficial, surely one must be open to the possibility that other benefits were involved. So how does one decide what benefits may flow from some social practice?

In 1848, Charles Simpson wrote a letter to the editor of *Lancet*; the letter contained this comment: "The history of the treatment of hydrophobia [i.e., rabies], tetanus, epilepsy, etc. is a greater reflection on the art and science of medicine than the inability to cure" (Simpson, 1848). In making this remark, Simpson was probably just objecting to the callousness of typical medical treatment in his day—an objection that may or may not have been warranted. However, his remark could also be taken to mean that *treatment*, that is, what physicians actually do, may be more revealing of what the medical profession is all about than whether physicians can successfully achieve their overt objective of controlling disease. On this reading, the quotation suggests this strategy: in trying to understand some system of medicine, it is not enough to consider only what physicians might *say* they are doing (e.g., seeking to reduce morbidity—the objective that the practitioners themselves or that we, as outside observers, might assume to be the goals of all medical practice); instead, one must carefully consider what physicians actually *do*. In the case of early nineteenth-century medicine, for example, one must consider bloodletting.

Of course, as in the case of the Lele villagers, the practitioners themselves may not have been aware of or even interested in the possibility that bloodletting achieved benefits beyond what could be seen as its strictly medical objectives. And even if they were, there may be little clear evidence of that awareness in the limited historical and anthropological materials available to us today—everything depends, after all, on what happens to have been recorded either in primary texts or in fieldworkers' interviews. However, even judging by the limited available evidence, aside from whatever benefits bloodletting may have had in reducing overall morbidity, the practice seems also to have had considerable social, moral, and psychological significance. These dimensions of bloodletting must also be taken into account in appraising the practice.

I

In the early nineteenth century, medical theory and practice were closely bound up with moral issues and with social roles. As we saw in chapter 1, William Buchan included "drinking spirituous liquors and [an] excess of venery" among the causes of ophthalmia. This is entirely typical. Etiological discussions of most diseases regularly included factors such as drunkenness, gluttony, indulgence, debauchery, dissipation, vicious habits, solitary vice, lustful excesses, indolence, sloth, envy, jealousy, and anger.[1] The specific choice of terms is important here—by identifying indolence (as opposed to inactivity), drunkenness (as opposed to intoxication), and solitary vice (as opposed to masturbation) in etiological discussions, moral concepts are invoked that permeate all subsequent theory and practice. If immorality is a cause of disease, the inculcation of traditional moral values becomes a treatment and a prophylaxis: "moderation in the pursuits of pleasure, of study, and of business; strict temperance and virtuous habits; may be said to comprise all that is most likely in our mode of living to give protection throughout life against the occurrence of scrofulous disease [a form of what is now called tuberculosis]" (Cumin, 1849, p. 140). "Few things are better preservatives against infection than fortitude and equanimity. Nothing, we are informed by those who voluntarily

31

exposed themselves to the contagion . . . was found [to be] so great a preservative against its effects, as a steady adherence to what they believed their duty, banishing from their minds . . . all thoughts of danger and avoiding every kind of passion" (Tweedie, 1849b, p. 177). Adherence to traditional moral standards was not only a protection against disease, it was also said to constitute the "most efficacious" part of therapy (Prichard, 1849a, p. 560). So how do these moral and social issues relate to bloodletting? To answer this question, we must understand more fully the conditions under which bloodletting was deemed to be an appropriate therapy.

As we saw in chapter 1, bloodletting was part of a general therapeutic approach called the antiphlogistic regimen. This approach seemed to be called for in at least *some* cases of virtually every disease, but it wasn't actually applied in *every* case of any disease. Given a disorder that involved fever or inflammation, how did physicians decide whether to invoke the antiphlogistic regimen? The choice of therapy was not determined merely by the diagnosis. Physicians criticized "writers of nosological systems" for believing that diagnosis alone could determine therapy—a belief that led physicians to prescribe "merely for a name" (Armstrong, 1825, p. 263). One physician explained that "there is no form of disease which, at all times, and under all circumstances, admits [of bloodletting], and . . . few which may not occasionally justify its use" (Clutterbuck, 1838b, p. 210). And the famous pathologist, Rudolf Virchow, observed that "Only the best physicians of all times have realized that similar cases of the most different diseases require the same treatment and that different cases of the same disease require different treatments. Conditions, rather than the disease, must be the basis for determination" (Virchow, 1856, p. 134). So what conditions determined whether to take blood?

In standard medical texts, in the discussions of almost every disease for which bloodletting is recommended, one encounters warnings of which the following two are typical:

> If there are clear indications that the hemorrhage is of an *active* or inflammatory character, venesection must be promptly resorted to, and followed up by purgatives and a strict antiphlogistic regimen. If, on the contrary, the disease puts on a *passive* or asthenic character, and the constitutional powers evince a tendency to sink rapidly, we must have early recourse to the most efficacious astringent remedies, and support the strength by mild but invigorating nourishment, and even cordials (Goldie, 1849, p. 360).

"In one case it may be necessary to bleed generally and locally—often to a considerable extent, . . . [while in other cases of the same disease] it may be necessary to administer nourishment and even stimulants . . . powerful cordials [may be] required to support the sinking powers" (Tweedie, 1849a, p. 103). As these warnings suggest, almost every disease could require diametrically opposed courses of treatment.

In deciding whether to adopt the antiphlogistic regimen, the crucial issue, as one physician observed, "is what is called, in common language, *fullness of habit*, or what we technically call *plethora* of the system" (Lawrence, 1829–30, p. 204). In a medical context, *plethora* meant literally a superabundance of blood; the term usually referred to an excess of blood in the entire system, but local inflammation could also be referred to as a local plethora. However, in contrast to inflammation, plethora itself was not regarded as a disease, and while it was often mentioned in etiological discussions, it was seldom identified as a cause of disease. Rather it seems most often to have been conceived of as a physical connection between such risk factors as gluttony, indolence, anger, or drunkenness—each of which seemed to produce at least a temporary excess of blood—and the symptoms or morbid lesions that constituted the disease. Thus, in the words of a contemporary physician, by means of the concept of plethora, "physiology becomes connected with pathology; the actual transition of health into disease is elucidated; and a light is thus shed on morbid processes which no other source of investigation can supply" (Barlow, 1849b, p. 553).

Thus, regardless of what disease had been diagnosed, the concept of plethora (fullness of habit) provided a basis for the selection of therapies, and it effectively divided the class of all patients into two subclasses, each member of either subclass requiring roughly the same treatment as any other member of the same subclass. Those who ate and drank too much, who were indolent, who had too much warmth, luxury, and sex, who thought too much or were too passionate, whose beds were too soft, or who took too many warm baths tended to become plethoric and to require bloodletting; those who ate too little, who labored in crowded factories, who had inadequate clothing and shelter, and who lacked fresh air became asthenic—the opposite of plethoric—and they required what was called supportive treatment.[1] As this suggests, membership in one or the other of these classes was determined by whether one's immoral acts or deviations from social norms were of a kind that involved excesses or deficiencies. In the etiological discussions in one medical encyclopedia, terms like "excessive diet," "gross and luxurious diet," "gluttony," "high feeding," and "full and stimulating diet" appear about four times as frequently as such terms as "insufficient food," or "want of stimulating diet" (Forbes, Tweedy, and Connolly). The prevalence of bleeding in early nineteenth-century medicine simply reflects the physicians' judgment that most people—at least most of those wealthy enough to seek help from regular practitioners—deviated from moral and social norms by way of excess rather than by way of deficiency. These observations reveal the nearly universal homeostatic model of disease. But here disease is construed not simply as a lack of equilibrium within the body—the level at which the model is most generally applied. Instead, or more accurately, in addition, the need for treatment here indicates that the patient is in disequilibrium with respect to *society*.

It can be no surprise that physicians occasionally let plethora (as well as the specific disease in question) fall from sight and simply concluded that wealth called for bleeding and poverty for supportive and tonic treatment. "It may be very well to bleed and otherwise re-duce those who have been well fed and have enjoyed all the comforts of life; but the practice is utterly inadmissible in a country where the poor are abandoned to a state of destitution, and, if not absolutely starved, are ill fed, and clothed, and lodged" (Jacob, 1849, p. 421). Another physician observed that scrofula (one form of what is now called tuberculosis) "is frequently engrafted on a feeble and attenu-ated frame; but it exists also in combination with a plethoric habit, . . . the first of these forms being often exemplified among the poor, the second among the rich . . . .. Hence, a broad line of distinction arises between the methods of treatment adapted to such different types of the disease" (Cumin, 1849, p. 140). The connection between wealth, in particular the abuses associated with wealth, and an excess of blood (plethora) was reflected in the ordinary speech of the day. The OED records that one use of the word *blood*, now obsolete, was as "'a hot spark,' 'a man of fire,' 'a buck,' a 'fast or foppish man,' 'a rake.'" The edi-tors observe that the term appears generally "to arise from the sense [of blood as] the supposed seat of emotions, passions, but in many cases also associated with [blood in the sense of] blood worth men-tioning, good blood, good parentage or stock [thus the term in this sense is equal to] an aristocratic rowdy." The OED cites uses of the word in this sense between 1562 and 1882. Suppose a *blood*, that is, an indolent, overeating, overdrinking, oversexed aristocrat, became ill; how should the physician have responded? Surely, the conceptual and semantic connections were too obvious to deny and too compelling to resist. Such excesses were virtually synonymous with plethora (fullness of habit, being a *blood*); and plethora led to illness. Removing blood reduced plethora—it compensated for the excesses; it restored the patient to the proper physiological, social, and moral balance; and it corrected what could otherwise have been a dangerous liability to disease. In such cases, the system of classification and the very terms that were used to mark the categories of treatment made it virtually impossible to deny that bloodletting was required.

David Wootton recounts the story of Antonio Durazzini who practiced medicine during a fever epidemic in a small town near Florence. According to Wootton, Durazzini treated those who could afford his services with the traditional remedies, especially bloodletting. Durazzini observed that "more of those who are able to seek medical advice and treatment die than of the poor," and Wootton speculates that Durazzini may have been unable or unwilling to recognize this result as a simple test of the effectiveness of medicine—perhaps, Wootton concludes, "he thought the poor were particularly robust" (Wootton, 2007, p. 140). But surely Durazzini would be more likely to have reported that the wealthy tended to be plethoric and, therefore, in more serious need of treatment. Later on Wootton observes that "early modern doctors only treated those who could afford to pay them. Vast numbers of people went without treatment, so that there would never have been any shortage of people to use as a control group had anyone wanted to compare the effects of treatment with no treatment" (Wootton, 2007, p. 145). But, even if they had thought in these terms (which they did not) from the point of view of early nineteenth-century physicians, this supposed control would have been totally inconclusive since, as we have seen, the rich were deemed plethoric and the poor not—so the disorders from which they suffered, regardless of the uniform diagnosis, were not thought to be the same.

Everyone seems to have been clear that *plethora* regularly preceded *illness* (but not necessarily the other way around—illness did not ordinarily produce plethora). But the connection between *immorality* and *plethora* seemed to operate in both directions: immorality (e.g., gluttony) could obviously bring on plethora, but plethora, in addition to endangering health, might also be conductive to deviant and rowdy behavior (to being a *blood*). Thus, "physicians employed the lancet as a moral prophylaxis for young [aristocratic] boys at the age of puberty. Bleeding was the 'best and only remedy for impulsive acts and eccentric emotions'; it removed many evils 'both moral and physical, which might otherwise damage the character and health very seriously'" (Haller, 1982, p. 51). So plethora threatened both health and morality. Not surprisingly, bloodletting seemed to be called for whenever one needed to restrain dangerous and unhealthy impulses: by removing blood one could cool the passions. One character in Flaubert's *Madame Bovary* observed, "If I were the government, I'd have all priests bled once a month. That's right . . . once a month! A nice big phlebotomy for the sake of public order and morality" (Flaubert, 1950, p. 67). And, in fact, in the fourteenth century, at the monastery at Barnwell, England, all "the monks were bled seven times a year, at Ely they were bled in weekly batches, each batch being about one-sixth of the convent. The Cistercians were bled in companies four times a year" (Flemming, 1957, p. 27). Thus, by correcting plethora, bleeding was deemed effective in fostering moral and regular behavior as well as good health.

Now we are in a position to identify some possible benefits to bloodletting beyond the mere control of inflammation and fever.

II

In discussing the classification schemes employed by various societies, Mary Douglas made this comment: "My wish has always been to take seriously [Emile] Durkheim's idea that the properties of classification systems derive from and are indeed properties of the social systems in which they are used" (Douglas, 1975, p. 296). It now appears that the basic scheme of classification by which early nineteenth-century physicians decided what therapy to invoke derived from and was, indeed, a property of the social system in which it was used. Selection of treatment had relatively little to do with the specific disease from which a patient was suffering; it had more to do with the socioeconomic class of a given patient. On the basis of his study of the medical systems of China, India, and the Arab World, Ivan Polunin observed that since "systems of medical practice have developed largely through interactions between sick persons and the people they consult, we might expect . . . that disease patterns have influenced the ways medical systems have evolved. My impression is that this has not been the case to any great extent" (Polunin, 1977). Our conclusions, based on early nineteenth-century bloodletting, may help explain Polunin's observation: perhaps earlier and non-Western medical systems, in general, have had little to do with disease except insofar as it provided leverage to reinforce morality and social norms.

Victor Turner has described the work of one *chimbuki* (which Turner translates as "doctor" although he points out that "'ritual specialist' or 'cult adept' would be equally appropriate") among the Ndembu, a tribe in Zambia. Turner concludes that the *chimbuki's* "main endeavor was to see that individuals were capable of playing their social roles successfully in a traditional structure of social position. Illness was for him a mark of undue deviation from the norm" (Turner, 1967, p. 392). Turner's observation applies perfectly in the context of early nineteenth-century medicine: there too illness was often a mark of deviation from the norm; there too practitioners were concerned with seeing that their patients returned to normal and traditional behavior. Because the term *chimbuki medicine* suggests clearly the application of a system of medicine in which, as among the Ndembu, the violation of norms was itself construed as a cause of disease and in which the practitioner sought to correct these violations, I prefer this term to *Hippocratic* or *traditional* medicine as a designation for what we are seeing in the early nineteenth century. However, it is important to understand that the essence of *chimbuki* medicine is *not* that the practitioner focused on moral and social issues *instead of* on morbidity and death. Rather, the point is that he focused on both at once or, more accurately, that *he focused on morality by way of morbidity*.

Was bloodletting actually effective as a means of reinforcing social and moral norms? This is an empirical question, and one that can probably never be conclusively answered. There is no way to examine past or non-Western societies to determine whether bloodletting—or the threat thereof—restrained people from disruptive behavior or whether it returned them to the norm in fact as well as symbolically. However, the willful disregard of social and moral norms can easily be more destructive of a society than is disease, and that being the case, one cannot simply dismiss a practice that involved reinforcing norms merely on the grounds that it does not produce what we would see as therapeutic benefits. It is entirely conceivable that chimbuki medicine was an effective tool in conserving moral and social order. This would help to explain how the practice of bloodletting could have been employed for centuries and virtually everywhere on earth even without yielding much beyond a placebo effect in regard to morbidity and mortality. It could also explain why non-Western systems of medicine seem to have no direct relation to the diseases that they have supposedly evolved to treat. Most importantly, for our purposes, it can also help us to see in therapeutic bloodletting something more than a colossal mistake.

However, in spite of helping us to understand some of the broader benefits that bloodletting may have contributed, so far our account is seriously incomplete. After mentioning a schizophrenic boy in Bruno Bettleheim's clinic who wanted to menstruate like adolescent girls, Mary Douglas observed that the boy wished to restore the "symmetry of his social world . . . by creating symmetry of the sexes within it" (Douglas, 1975, p. 71). We have seen that one benefit that may have been achieved by the system of classifications of early nineteenth-century medicine was the conservation of traditional social norms—one could say that by bleeding the rich and by supporting the poor, nineteenth-century physicians sought to restore the symmetry of their social world by creating symmetry of the classes within it. However, given that patients presumably found bleeding distasteful, one might well doubt whether their sense of a need to symbolically transcend their class distinctions could itself have provided sufficient pressure to maintain the practice. As George A. De Vos observed about one of the tribes mentioned by Douglas, "one could easily argue that the Australians might find a less bloody and potentially traumatic way to represent their social bifurcation" than by splitting the urethra of a pubescent boy with a sharpened stone (De Vos, 1975, p. 79). And Douglas herself pointed out that no system of classification can command general acceptance without supporting pressures from within the society itself—pressures that arise from the otherwise unsatisfied needs of individuals within the society (Douglas, 1975, p. 217). Social explanations of widely held theories are often incomplete without an account of the psychological benefits that provide pressure to maintain those theories. What one requires, therefore, is an explanation of how the practice of bloodletting achieved psychological benefits for individual patients.

An important clue as to the form this explanation will take is given by a rather remarkable triad of parallels that was frequently invoked by early nineteenth-century practitioners: first, physicians frequently assumed that *bloodletting* was an artificial substitute for *menstruation*. For example, one often finds passages such as this:

> A tendency of plethora in the head will be best counteracted by occasional revulsive bleeding from the lower extremities: as, for instance, the abstraction of a few ounces of blood from the feet . . ..

> We have found this plan particularly useful in cases of suppressed or irregular menstruation, and by having recourse to it at the approach of the menstrual period, or on the first appearance of any of the symptoms threatening an attack of convulsions, we may often succeed in warding it off. (Crawford, 1849, p. 518)

Second, physicians at the time regarded *hemorrhoidal* bleeding, especially in males, as a beneficial equivalent to *menstruation*. This entailed that bloodletting was an artificial substitute for either. For example, in etiological discussions, one frequently finds specific diseases ascribed to "the suppression of habitual discharges, such as hemorrhoidal and menstrual flux" (Townsend, 1849, p. 159). Here are three passages, taken almost at random from a virtually unlimited number that further illustrate these connections:

> Should a suppression of the hemorrhoidal discharge be the cause [of a case of hemoptysis], aloetic purgatives, and leeches applied *circa anum*, are the means to be employed. If the suspended menstrual discharge seems to be the cause . . . we try to assist the abortive efforts of nature at the ordinary period of the menstrual discharge, by determining [blood] to the uterus by means of aloetic purgatives, [and] by leeches applied to the interior of the thighs (Law, 1849, p. 369).
>
> When habitual discharges from the hemorrhoidal veins have been coerced [to stop], or have ceased spontaneously, derangement of the health has ensued similar to that occasioned by uterine suppressions . . . [in one case] paralysis became complicated with madness in consequence of the suppression of a habitual hemorrhoidal discharge. The application of a single leech to the hemorrhoidal veins every day during the month was followed by a restoration of the flux, and the patient was cured of his complaint (Prichard, 1849b, p. 62).
>
> Hoffman describes the case of a woman, thirty years of age, previously strong and healthy, in whom the menstrual discharge was in general remarkably copious. Having suffered from a fright immediately before the menstrual period, the discharge did not take place, and she was seized with languor, loss of appetite, and dropsical swelling to such a degree that the integuments on the feet burst and discharged serum in great quantity. The menstrual discharge having taken place at the next period, all these complaints were removed . . . .. Similar symptoms have been occasionally observed in connection with suppression of hemorrhoidal discharge after it has become habitual . . . .. Bloodletting is the first remedy demanded, and in almost every case this should be general [bloodletting] (Darwell, 1849, p. 98).

Early nineteenth-century physicians were not the first to regard bloodletting as an artificial parallel to menstruation and to hemorrhoidal bleeding: Galen took the same position centuries earlier. The following passage is from Galen's tract entitled "On Venesection against Erasistratus" in which he supports bloodletting and argues against Erasistratus, who had challenged some uses of the practice:

> It is necessary, in my opinion, that the female sex, who stay indoors, neither engaging in strenuous labor nor exposing themselves to direct sunlight—both factors conducive to the development of plethos—should have a natural remedy [i.e., menstruation] by which it is evacuated. This is one of the ways in which nature operates in these conditions; another is the cleansing that follows childbirth . . . . A woman does not suffer from gout, says Hippocrates, unless her menses fail. Yet why bother to quote Hippocrates to [Erasistratus], a man who is hostile to him? I see myself rather as a town crier shouting the truth at you, that a woman who is well cleansed is not seized with gouty or arthritic or pleuritic or peripneumonic diseases, and that neither epilepsy nor apoplexy or suspension of breathing nor loss of speech occur at any time if she is properly cleansed. Has a woman ever been known to be stricken with phrenitis, or lethargy, or spasm, or tremor, or tetany, while her menstrual periods were coming? Or did you ever hear of a woman who suffered from melancholy or madness of haemoptysis or haematemesis, or headache, or suffocation from synanche, or from any of the major and severe diseases, if her menstrual secretions were well established? And, on the other hand, if they are suppressed, she is certain to fall into every sort of illness. Thus even evacuations are healing remedies. But enough of women for the present; come now to consider the men, and learn how those who eliminate the excess through a haemorrhoid all pass their lives unaffected by diseases, while those in whom the evacuations have been restrained have fallen into the gravest illnesses. Will you not let blood from these men, even if they become synanchic or peripneumonic? . . . I, on the other hand, have often cured, not only these conditions, but even spasm and dropsy, by the removal of blood . . .
>
> Do not suppose, therefore, that your quarrel is with Hippocrates alone when he recommends the evacuation of blood, in cases where a man, through suppression of a haemorrhoid, or a woman, from suppression of the menses, falls into a rigor, or a dropsy, or any other cold disease; you are at odds too with all physicians who rely on experience, and with the life of man, for you seem to me to be overturning the common doctrine of all of them. Would you not concede that the natural course anyone would take when faced with a plethos of blood was to evacuate it? Who does not know that opposites are the cure for opposites? This is not the

doctrine of Hippocrates alone; it is the common belief of all men. (Brain, 1986, p. 26f)

Today, it may seem very odd that anyone could regard menstruation, male haemorrhoidal bleeding, and bloodletting as more or less parallel to one another. The frequent appeal to these associations in early nineteenth-century medical writings and the fact that the associations go back as far as Galen cry out for an explanation more deeply rooted in the human psyche than the mere desire for therapy. But the need for such an explanation becomes absolutely compelling only with the discovery that strikingly similar parallels have been documented, in our own times, in the medical thinking of various remote cultures. For example, Bruno Bettleheim notes that "Wogeo men of New Guinea say that women are automatically cleansed by menstruation, but that men, to guard against illness, periodically incise the penis and allow some blood to flow; an operation which is often called 'men's menstruation'" (Bettelheim, 1962, p. 19). More recently, Leonard B. Glick has described similar rituals among the Gimi, another tribe in New Guinea (Glick, 1967, p. 50). As both Bettelheim and Glick point out, these pseudomenstrual rituals are explained as health-promoting practices that can be beneficial for all the adult men in the community. One must wonder what is going on here. The psychologists have provided what may be a partial explanation.

Bettelheim sought to explain primitive initiation rites with the supposition that "one sex feels envy in regard to the sexual organs and functions of the other" (Bettelheim, 1962, p. 19). He discussed various societies in which initiation rites enabled the adolescent "to master his [or her] envy of the other sex, or to adjust to the social role prescribed for his [or her] sex." He observed that in such societies, the rituals for girls differ from those for boys by involving manipulation of the initiant's genitals by both men and women rather than exclusively by members of the same sex. Moreover, in the rites for girls, the "manipulation by men is destructive, showing an aggressive enmity that is most readily explained by fear or envy." For boys, initiation usually involved circumcision, subincision, and even certain ritual practices supposedly to control defecation. Many of these rites were intentionally and admittedly patterned after specific female functions such as menstruation and delivery.

According to Bettelheim, the object of all these rites is to help the initiant accept the natural inevitability of being limited to one sex and to identify the initiant as an active participant in the social role of that sex. Similarly, Leonard B. Glick observes that "in drawing blood from their noses and forearms, men . . . imitate women, paradoxically transcending their maleness and at the same time guaranteeing its perpetuation" (Glick, 1967, p. 50). There is another possible aspect to male bleeding that conforms well with Bettelheim's thesis but that neither he nor Glick mentions: one token of wealth has always been conspicuous disbursement either by consumption, by the bestowal of gifts, or simply by the destruction of valuable property. What better token could there be of a man's superior endowment of vitality, life, and power than his ability to withstand, voluntarily, more frequent and more extensive losses of blood than nature extracts from women? Thus, in being bled, in dispersing the essence of life itself, the masculinity and the superiority of the male was reaffirmed.

Now all of this is obviously and strikingly parallel to what we found in early nineteenth-century medicine: physicians guarded against illness by periodically drawing blood from male aristo-crats. Of course, women were also bled, but much less frequently than men because, as the physicians themselves explained, women achieved the same beneficial cleansing through natural menstrua-tion that men could achieve only through hemorrhoidal discharges or through artificial bleeding. Recent studies show clearly enough that the aggression Bettelheim detected in male contributions to the girls' initiation rites had a counterpart in the treatment of women by nineteenth-century practitioners (Shorter, 1980). Given these paral-lels, if Bettelheim is more or less correct, his theory may also reveal some psychological benefits to nineteenth-century bleeding. Male bleeding, like the bold and risky behavior typical of males everywhere and always, may have been a way of demonstrating male toughness and superiority.

The early decades of the nineteenth century, the decades that culminated in the revolutions of 1848, were a period of social stress. Industrialization exaggerated the disparity between social extremes; the emergence of the middle class threatened the entire traditional social structure. Under these conditions, one might expect nineteenth-century physicians to reassure aristocratic patients about the value of their traditional roles and to provide a means for them to demonstrate their power and significance. As the aristocracy lost hegemony, the physician might have been expected to provide a means of reaffirming masculinity and superiority and, at the same time, of guaranteeing the perpetuation of both. Let us suppose that Bettelheim is approximately correct in his interpretation of the initiation rites. Bloodletting could have provided roughly similar psychological benefits that parallel rites seem to have provided in other societies when social and sexual roles need to be adopted or reconfirmed. In the face of ambiguity, bleeding may have reaffirmed one's masculinity and superiority and redefined one's relation to women and to members of the lower social orders, none of whom were bled nearly so frequently as *bloods*—as young male aristocrats. This, too, could have been a benefit derived from bloodletting, a psychological benefit to the individual and one that helped provided the pressure to maintain a practice that, on the social level, compensated for class disequilibrium.

III

We must consider one final dimension of nineteenth-century bloodletting. Mary Douglas observed that "whenever the organic erupts into the social, there is impurity; birth, death, sex, eating, and defecation incur impurity, and so are hedged with rituals" (Douglas, 1975, p. 214). Douglas did not mention disease, but surely disease is as much an organic disruption of the social as any of the phenomena she lists. So here, too, we must expect, not just treatment, but ritual. The distinguished American historian of medicine Charles E. Rosenberg acknowledges that much of earlier medical treatment was ritualistic, but he goes one step further in connecting the medical rituals specifically to religion. He has suggested that the use of strong drugs such as mercury, antimony, and arsenic, which were important in the so-called heroic treatment that characterized the early nineteenth century, had *religious* overtones. In discussing some of the terms that were used to describe the therapeutic interaction between physicians and patients, he notes that exhibiting a drug was synonymous with administering it. He then observes that

> the therapeutic interaction . . . was a fundamental cultural ritual, in a literal sense . . . .. To "exhibit" a drug was to act out a sacramental role in the liturgy of healing. The analogy to religious ritual is not exact, but it is certainly more than metaphorical. A sacrament, after all, is conventionally defined as an external, visible symbol of an invisible, internal state. Insofar as a particular drug caused a perceptible physiological effect, it produced phenomena which all—the physician, the patient, and the patient's family—could witness (again the double meaning, with its theological overtones is instructive), and in which all could participate (Rosenberg, 1979, p. 10).

If Rosenberg is correct in finding a religious significance in the administration of powerful drugs, by so much the more must this be true of *bloodletting*—the shedding of innocent blood, the shedding of the essence of life. The parallels are obvious and striking: in bloodletting, members of a kind of priesthood, all of whom were necessarily male, all of whom had taken vows that bound them to their profession and to one another, all of whom diagnosed and prescribed in the official language of the Church (a language largely unknown to laymen), mediated what can be described, literally, as an atonement by blood—an atonement in the sense that the patient was again made *one* with those who had not violated the norms. In the great nineteenth-century pseudomenstrual rite, by being bled—by voluntarily and liberally disbursing the essence of his own life—the threatened aristocrat paid the price for sin, he paid the price for the personal and social disequilibrium created by his own excessive wealth, power, and consumption, and, at the same time, by demonstrating his strength and power, he was reconfirmed in the social and familial role that warranted those excesses. By voluntarily laying down his life, he was justified in taking it up again. The external and visible symbol of bloodletting produced and guaranteed continuation of the *internal* yet equally *visible* state of health and dominion. Expiation and justification were wrought, literally, by the shedding of blood.

So what are we now to conclude about bloodletting and about chimbuki medicine in general? We see that, beyond its use in reducing inflammation, bloodletting may have provided social, moral, and psychological benefits within the societies in which it was practiced. In discussing the rising fertility rates in the eighteenth and nineteenth centuries, David Wootton points out that "in the early modern period fertility was kept in check by deliberate abstinence on the part of the unmarried, and . . . in the eighteenth and nineteenth centuries abstinence became much less popular. In short, people became more sexually active. There is no adequate study of why this might be, but a reasonable guess is that it reflects the decline in the church courts and of other mechanisms, formal and informal, of policing sexual behavior" (Wootton, 2007, p. 276). And, if Wootton is right, it is equally reasonable to suppose that among these informal mechanisms was chimbuki medicine. Of course, we cannot conclude that this was a goal (conscious or otherwise) in every society in which blood was taken, or even that in those societies where such benefits were realized, everyone who participated in the practice, either as physicians or as patients, thought in these terms. Nevertheless, the fragmentary evidence that we can weave together is richly suggestive. Clearly, in appraising bloodletting, more must be taken into account than simply the reduction of morbidity and the prolongation of life.

Indeed, we can state the point somewhat more strongly. Suppose we insist that chimbuki medicine was *bad* medicine because, after all, it did not significantly prolong life or reduce morbidity. Surely early nineteenth-century physicians could level the same accusation against us because of our total indifference to the moral and social lives of our patients and to the integrity of the society in which we live—indifference to the goals that seem to have informed their practice. Our indifference to these issues would be something that earlier physicians might have found shocking, appalling—at least as shocking as we find their wholesale use of bloodletting. Suppose (one might object on behalf of an earlier physician) physicians of the twenty-first century enable persons to live a few extra years but at the cost of consigning them to decaying and dysfunctional neighborhoods where they are constantly confronted by drug abuse and street crime; is extending life under these conditions sufficient to insure that we are finally practicing *good* medicine? All things taken into account, might it not be better to adopt a medical system that seeks, at least, to address some of these broader problems? Of course, it would be impossible to return to an earlier system even if it were clear that it would be desirable to do so (which it definitely is not). My only point is that a simple comparison of mortality rates cannot tell us who is practicing good medicine—the issue is far too complicated for that to be possible.

But what of the medical system in which bloodletting was the central therapy? If the primary benefits of bloodletting were moral and psychological, must not this also be reflected throughout the entire medical system to which bloodletting was so crucial? And if so, must we not expect that that medical system will bear marks of this association? As we will see in the next two chapters, there is collateral evidence that this was, indeed, the case.

Note

1.   These factors are mentioned in various essays in Forbes, Tweedie, and Conolly (1832–5).

3

Disease and Causes of Disease in Early Nineteenth-Century Medical Thought

In general, to ensure that something will happen, we look for a
sufficient cause; to insure that something will not happen, we look for
a necessary cause.
—K. Codell Carter (2005)

Don't go out without your coat on, you'll catch cold.

In 1845 James L. Bardsley, a prominent British physician, wrote that diabetes "has been traced by some patients to sleeping out the whole of the night in a state of intoxication" (Bardsley, 1849, p. 609). This statement seems curious not simply because Bardsley identified a cause that we no longer find plausible; more fundamental issues are involved. For one thing, Bardsley assumed that patients' opinions could be important or even decisive in identifying the causes of their illnesses. And this assumption, in turn, raises the possibility that different cases of the same disorder could have entirely different causes. What are we to make of these assumptions?

In the same year that Bardsley wrote about diabetes, Wilhelm Friedrich Scanzoni, director of the Prague maternity clinic, proposed to study the etiology of childbed fever, an often fatal disease that struck women a day or two after child birth. As part of his study, Scanzoni urged the authorities to require local physicians to report each case of childbed fever that occurred in their practices. In their reports, they were to give "particular attention to the causal factors of the disease" (Scanzoni, 1850, p. 32). Scanzoni intended to study the etiology of childbed fever by determining the frequency of the different causes to which local physicians ascribed individual cases. Like Bardsley, Scanzoni assumed that different cases of a given disease could have completely different causes and that a list of these causes could be compiled simply by looking at one case after another.

Contemporary medical texts contain the results of surveys like the one Scanzoni proposed to conduct. Seven years earlier, A.E. Chomel, a leading French internist, explained that one could investigate the causes of pneumonia "by interrogating carefully a certain number of individuals struck by this affliction, and by directing one's questions to the causes that produced it" (Chomel, 1838, p. 165f). In his own study, "made with great care on seventy-nine pneumonia patients," he found the following: fourteen patients reported experiencing some form of cooling, five had consumed too much wine, two had worked excessively, one had experienced a lively emotion, and another had inhaled carbon vapor. The fifty-six remaining patients were unable to explain how they had become ill. Chomel also reported an earlier study of 125 patients in which the following causes had been established: contusions of the throat, two; cooling, thirty-eight; violent effort and fatigue, twelve; depression, four; excess of drink or upset regimen, three; and in the remaining sixty-six cases, no cause could be identified.

Proceeding in this case-by-case way, physicians accumulated extensive lists of possible causes for each disease. For example, in his account of diabetes, Bardsley identified the following causes: frequent exposure to sudden alterations of heat and cold, indulgence in copious draughts of cold fluid when the system has been overheated by labor or exercise, intemperate use of spirituous liquors, poor living, sleeping out the whole of the night in the open air in a state of intoxication, checking perspiration suddenly, and mental anxiety and distress (Bardsley, 1849, p. 609). This, no doubt, was also the general approach that led to William Buchan's list of possible causes of ophthalmia that we encountered in chapter 1. And similar lists can be found for virtually any disease in most German, English, or French medical texts from the period. How are we to understand these lists of causes?

I

Causal concepts are rooted in everyday interests in controlling and understanding the world. Our interests vary, and so does our language about causes. We talk about causes of individual events (what caused the accident) and of classes of events (what causes lightening); we use causes to explain what has happened in the past or is happening now (what caused the power failure) and to predict what will happen in the future (will adding iron to the soil cause the leaves to become darker green); we seek causes to insure that events will happen (what will cause the oil slick to dissipate) and to prevent events from happening (what will cause the window to stop sticking). The terms *necessary* and *sufficient* mark two broad kinds of causes both of which interest us in daily life. In general, to explain why some event or class of events happens or to insure or predict that such events will happen, we look for a cause whose occurrence will be accompanied by the event—that is we look for a sufficient cause. However, when we want to explain why some event or class of events doesn't happen or to insure or to predict that such events won't happen, we look for a cause whose absence will be accompanied by the absence of the event—that is we look for a necessary cause. So, depending on our interests, we sometimes seek sufficient and sometimes necessary causes. Because our interests in the two kinds of causes are different, the causes in these two classes are usually also different: most causes are not both necessary and sufficient. For example, a cause of death is usually a sufficient cause of a single event (it explains why one person died), but it is not usually necessary (something else could also have caused the person to die). One exception is lightening which is both sufficient and necessary for thunder.

What sorts of causes were identified in early nineteenth-century practical medicine? What was the relation between some particular cause, say anxiety, and the disease that was, supposedly, its effect? Clearly, no one cause was *necessary* for the onset of any specific disease since, as we have seen, different cases of each disease were ascribed to a range of different causes. One person contracted diabetes because of anxiety, but this wasn't necessary—he could just as well have become diabetic after spending the night outside while intoxicated. Physicians explicitly denied that the same cause was present in every case of any disease: "No inference can fairly be drawn from the identity of the effect, for certain diseased states are produced by a variety of remote causes, this expression being used in the sense usually annexed to it by medical men" (Brown, 1849, p. 505). However, particular causes seem not to have been thought of as *sufficient* either. A typical factor, say anxiety, could be listed as a possible cause for many different diseases. For example, one widely used British medical encyclopedia identified anxiety as a possible cause of dozens of diseases including acne, catalepsy, diabetes, ecthyma, fever, herpes, hydrocephalus, impetigo, senile dementia, psoriasis, scrofula, and tetanus (Forbes, Tweedie, and Conolly, 1849). Thus, anxiety was not expected always to result in the same disease—one anxious person might become diabetic but others might contract impetigo or tetanus. So, strictly speaking, causes were not sufficient either.

However, while individual causes were not thought of as sufficient, they could be part of a combination of factors that, as a whole, *was* sufficient. To understand this, we must take account of another distinction that was important in nineteenth-century etiology. Causes were generally classified as *predisposing* or *exciting*. (Exciting causes were sometimes referred to as *occasioning*.) Predisposing causes "render the body liable to become the prey of something, which has a tendency to excite the disease. The exciting [or occasioning] cause of the disease might have no effect, unless the body had been predisposed; and the predisposition might not have had the effect, unless the exciting cause had occurred" (Elliotson, 1844, p. 43). Typically, any account of a disease would include both predisposing and exciting causes. For example, one discussion of tetanus mentioned these predisposing causes: warm climate, humid situations, bad or insufficient nutriment, close and ill-ventilated habitations, inattention to cleanliness, and neglect of the bowels; the same discussion listed these exciting causes: mechanical wounds, application of cold and damp, the irritation of worms, terror, sympathy, mental anguish, the suppression of perspiration, the accumulation of cherry-stones in the intestines, suppression of lochia, and gastric inflammation (Symonds, 1849, p. 368). Contemporary writers observed that, if allowed to persist over time, predisposing causes could themselves become exciting and that under some circumstances, what were usually exciting causes could function as predisposing causes (Elliotson, 1844, p. 45). Moreover under suitable circumstances, either kind of cause alone could bring on a disease (Conolly, 1849, p. 678). One writer observed that "the same occasional cause can provoke the development of all the diseases, and the same disease can be created by every kind of occasioning cause" (Chomel, 1838, p. 425). If a typical cause is neither necessary nor sufficient, how can distinguishing between predisposing and exciting causes help provide a complete sufficient causal explanation for the onset of a disease?

Several discussions of disease causation include some version of this hypothetical case:

> Of several individuals exposed to the same exciting cause, scarcely two will be affected alike. From exposure to cold, for instance, one will be attacked with catarrh, another with rheumatism, a third with

inflammation of the bowels, a fourth with sore throat; while by far the greater number will escape altogether. Were the exciting cause solely chargeable with these several effects, they would unquestionably be marked with greater uniformity. The truth is, that the exciting cause produces its effect because the body exposed to it is prone to be morbidly affected in consequence of its own previous derangement; and the specific form of the disease is determined, partly by the operation of the exciting cause, but chiefly by the predisposition of the parts affected to undergo those morbid actions to which the general indisposition of the system and their own partial weakness render them liable. (Barlow, 1849b, p. 555)

Thus, it was believed that, with the help of other predisposing and exciting factors, any single cause could, in principle, be filled out into a fully sufficient explanation of the onset of an illness. For example, in 1835, while explaining why different persons react differently when exposed to a cold damp wind, a French writer observed that "this experiment proves only that which observation confirms every day, namely, that the same cause can give rise to different effects, according to the particular state of the individual on which it acts. Thus the same frozen drink given to several perspiring persons produces in one a simple loss of voice, in another a cold, in a third a very serious laryngitis, etc." (Trousseau, 1835, p. 338). Fourteen years later, another French physician wrote that no one could predict what would happen when persons were exposed to a particular exciting cause, say, sudden chilling—some become rheumatic, some develop pulmonary catarrh or diarrhea, and others remains healthy. He then observed that "a previous examination of each [victim] would no doubt solve the problem" (Lagasquie, 1849, p. 313). Of course, in practice, no examination could be thorough enough to identify all the relevant "indispositions and partial weaknesses" and thereby enable one to predict the exact outcome of some new trauma. However, in principle, the collection of all the causes—both predisposing and exciting—would be sufficient for the particular effect. Moreover, presumably, any two persons affected by precisely the same set of predisposing and exciting causes would suffer the same effect.

All of this suggests that a single cause, such as those identified at the beginning of this chapter, could be any trauma that seemed especially striking to the patient or to the physician and that seemed as though it could plausibly help explain the onset of one case of the disease. Such a cause was thought of as one part of a combination of conditions that, collectively, constituted a sufficient cause for that particular instance of disease. There is nothing unreasonable about such causal explanations: they are almost exactly what one would look for, today, if one were interested in explaining why some individual became ill. It was also reasonable to think that patients could be aware of salient traumata that might be part of such an explanation. From our point of view, no less than from that of nineteenth-century physicians, experiences that patients report, experiences such as overexertion, sleep deprivation, or poor diet, could be part of a sufficient explanation of the onset of a particular case of illness. This is how one must understand Bardsley's comment that some patients had traced illness to "sleeping out the whole of the night in a state of intoxication." Understood in this way, the claim is at least reasonable if no longer entirely plausible.

However, we are now prepared to appreciate one striking difference between early nineteenth-century discussions of etiology and those in our own day: both in ordinary everyday conversation and in technical medical discourse, we today speak of "*the* cause of X," where X is the name of some disease; for example, "the cause of diabetes" or "the cause of tuberculosis." When we speak in this way, we are not interested in how some individual contracted the disease but, rather, in some common factor or set of factors that enters into every case of the disease. If we ask: "what is the cause of AIDS?" we are not usually interested in being told that person A contracted AIDS by using an infected hypodermic needle and that person B contracted it by practicing unprotected sex. Instead, we are seeking something like HIV which is common to all cases of AIDS. By contrast, in the earlier literature, one looks in vain for any talk of "*the* cause of disease X." Among causes, one finds only the sets of exciting and predisposing causes of individual cases such as those we have listed and characterized. One reason for the apparent strangeness of James L. Bardsley's account of the causes of diabetes is that, in such a discussion, we would now expect an account of *the* cause of diabetes (so far as it is understood) not just a list of factors deemed to have contributed to certain individuals becoming diabetic. But in the early 1800s, there were no such accounts; there simply was no concept of "the cause of disease X." Why might this have been?

One reason is this: given how diseases were then defined, it was reasonable and virtually inevitable that different episodes of any disease would be attributed to a variety of unrelated causes. As we have seen, in the early nineteenth century, diseases were almost always characterized as one or more disordered states—some condition or set of conditions that would be apparent both to the patient and to the physician. For example, in a lecture delivered at the University of Paris in 1832 and reprinted in the British journal, *Lancet*, Gabriel Andral defined "hydrophobia" (which would now be called rabies) as "complete horror of fluids, reaching to such a degree, that their deglutition becomes almost impossible" (Andral, 1832–3, p. 806). Thus, *hydrophobia* was defined in terms of one prominent anomaly: an extreme inability to swallow. However, if hydrophobia is a horror of swallowing, then, as Andral willingly acknowledged, fully authentic cases could be caused by blows to the throat or by psychological problems as well as by the bites of rabid dogs. Given a definition like Andral's, it was logical and inevitable that hydrophobia, or any other disease so defined, would be thought of as having a range of different possible remote causes. Similarly, if we define *diabetes* as voiding a disproportionate quantity of water, then it can indeed be brought on by various factors such as by drinking too much cider or by overwork. And, of course, this is just what we saw in William Buchan's account of ophthalmia. So it is not simply that earlier physicians failed to notice a commonality among the causes of individual cases, a commonality that we have since managed to discern. Given contemporary characterizations of diseases in terms of physical anomalies, there was no commonality: within their system of ideas, the phrase "the cause of disease X" could have no meaning.

There are ways of characterizing diseases other than in terms of overt physical dysfunctions. In the early nineteenth century, phthisis, a prominent disease at the time, was characterized as coughing so intensely that it involved spitting up blood—a condition that, like most other disordered states, could be caused in many different ways. However, anatomical studies revealed that these physical conditions were often associated with distinctive caseating tumors or tubers in the lungs—a condition called tuberculosis. At the beginning of the century, phthisis and tuberculosis were usually regarded as distinct conditions because each was known to occur without the other. However, when phthisis symptoms and tubers occurred together, the tubers seemed to explain the symptoms, and phthisis could be regarded as a particular manifestation or development of tuberculosis. Johann Lucas Schönlein, a prominent German pathologist, wrote: "In recent times phthisis has been regarded, not as a unique disease, but as a direct sequel and higher development of tuberculosis. This opinion arose first in [Marie-Francois-Xavier] Bichat's school and has spread through France, England, and even part of Germany" (Schönlein, 1832, p. 134). Schönlein did not himself agree with this way of thinking; he objected on the grounds that some genuine cases of phthisis did not involve tubers. However, he admitted, "One cannot deny credit to the pathologists who have provided this material basis for phthisis." By providing a "material basis," the pathologists explained the overt physical dysfunctions and made diagnosis more reliable and precise. For these reasons, and because it seemed so enlightening, phthisis was ultimately recharacterized in terms of tubers; nontuberous cases, which had formerly been genuine instances of phthisis, were reclassified simply as intense coughing but were no longer called phthisis.

Because the new characterization of phthisis seemed superior and because, at the time, phthisis was such a prominent disease, this approach became a model for characterizing other diseases. Physicians dissected corpses, sought morbid remains, and, when possible, redefined diseases in terms of what they found. The new characterizations were recognized as important advances. "The great improvements which have taken place of late years in pathology, by enabling practitioners to connect symptoms with their organic causes more accurately, have necessarily diverted attention from the artificial [merely symptomatic] combinations of the old nosology" (Forbes, 1849, p. 106).

However, the influence of pathological anatomy went further than just providing new ways of defining diseases. Thomas Watson began a lecture on morbid anatomy by stressing that "the topic is not one of merely curious interest, but has a direct bearing upon the proper treatment of diseases. It teaches us what we have to guard against, what we must strive to avert, in different cases. In speaking of particular diseases, I shall constantly refer to the facts and reasonings which I am now about to lay before you" (Watson, 1858, p. 68). Thus, the examination of corpses became a major source of knowledge about the proper and improper functioning of the body—about health and disease. By following this model, physicians were inevitably influenced not only by the content—the specific observations and explanations—but also by the *form* of the explanations that pathologists provided.

Of what form were the causes that interested pathologists? The causes pathologists identified (and that physicians took as a basis for their "facts and reasonings" about diseases) were causes of death and causes of the successive stages of morbid processes. It was natural to associate causes of disease with causes of death. Indeed, it could not have been otherwise: whenever possible, diseases were defined as morbid processes, and unchecked morbid processes end in death. Thus, in contemporary medical texts, the discussion of individual diseases was often immediately preceded by a discussion of causes of death (e.g., Watson, 1858, pp. 67–70). But a cause of death or the cause of a certain morbid alteration, like the cause of an accident or of the malfunction of a watch, is a sufficient cause for a particular event; one is asking, "Why did this person die now?" And this, by the way, is no less true today than it was two hundred years ago—the causes of death that we, today, identify are exactly of this form (King, 1982, p. 213). From their symptomatically oriented predecessors, anatomically oriented pathologists inherited a preoccupation with sufficient causes for particular events; the fascination with pathology only reinforced this preoccupation. Thus, causal thinking in medicine was almost unaffected by the change from symptomatic to anatomical characterizations of diseases. The lists of remote causes of diseases that we considered at the beginning of this chapter spanned, essentially unchanged, the shift from symptomatic to anatomical characterizations.

Insofar as one is interested in explaining why an individual becomes sick or dies, it is (from our point of view, no less than from that of a nineteenth-century physician) logical and correct to look for a sufficient cause for that single event and such a cause would, still today, inevitably include a variety of what could be called predisposing and exciting factors. However, in the early nineteenth century, given symptomatic or anatomical characterizations of diseases, there was simply no other way of thinking about causes. And, assuming one is limited to causes of this kind, the nearest one could come to our concept of "the cause of disease X" would be a sort of compilation of different causes found in individual cases—just the sort of collection that Scanzoni, Chomel, and Buchan identified in their accounts of childbed fever, pneumonia, and ophthalmia, respectively. Thus, in these decades, physicians focused on a kind of cause—sufficient causes for particular events—that receives relatively little medical attention today, while causes of the sort that dominate our etiological thinking—universal necessary causes—were virtually absent.

However, medical focus exclusively on this kind of cause is more curious than one might at first realize, and here is the reason: one normally looks for a *sufficient* cause if one wants to bring about some state of affairs, say pneumonia in a test animal, but if one wants to avoid that disease, one looks for a *necessary* cause (Carter, 2005, p. 432). This is because, by avoiding a necessary cause, one can be sure that one will not contract the disease. Finding sufficient causes—such causes as we might now classify as risk factors—can sometimes help in controlling disease, but they can never be as effective as necessary causes. Yet before the middle of the nineteenth century, physicians were interested almost exclusively in sufficient causes. Thus, earlier medical thinking about causes simply did not line up with the supposed goal of preventing or curing disease. To prevent disease, one would like to have pointed out that physicians should have been looking for necessary causes. How could earlier physicians—physicians who were, presumably, interested in diminishing morbidity and disease— have become preoccupied with a kind of cause that can insure that some effect will occur, but that is of much less significance when it comes to insuring that it will not? How could such a preoccupation have persisted literally for millennia? Did such causes serve some other purpose? To help understand this situation, we must consider one further aspect of early nineteenth-century etiology, and here the insights of anthropologists become relevant.

II

As we have seen, nineteenth-century physicians were more inter-ested in questions like "Why does this person now have mumps?" than in questions like "How does mumps come about?" Exactly the same priority of interests has been repeatedly noted in explanations of misfortune in non-Western societies, and, as various anthropolo-gists have independently concluded, the reason is always the same: the primary objective is not controlling or even explaining misfortune, but reinforcing norms (Evans-Pritchard, 1976, pp. 19–23; Foster, 1965; Frankfurt et al., 1949, p. 25). In addressing the same issue from a slightly different perspective, Mary Douglas drew attention to the frequency with which conformity is encouraged (both in non-Western cultures and in our own) by portraying deviancy as a threat to such assets as time, money, nature, or divine favor (Douglas, 1975, pp. 230–48). Here again, misfortune, or the threat of potential misfortune, is held up as a way of securing conformity. Douglas does not mention *health* as one such asset but, clearly, endangerment of health is frequently used for the same purpose. We try to prevent behavior of which we disapprove by portraying it as unhealthy: "Don't go out without your coat on, you will catch cold," "Don't drink soda drinks, they are bad for your teeth," "Don't smoke, it causes cancer," "Don't masturbate, you may go blind." Representing some behavior as sufficient to bring on disease is a natural, almost universally espoused, and (possibly) even mildly effective way to influence behavior. What must we conclude about any set of physicians who are exclusively interested in sufficient causes for particular cases of disease and, indeed, in causes many of which turn out to be violations of social and moral norms?

We have seen that moral considerations were important in early nineteenth-century etiology—moral transgressions were regularly identified as actual causes of disease. Among the causes of disease that were identified in typical etiological discussions from the period, one finds such factors as the following: drunkenness, intemperance, gluttony, luxury, indulgence, debauchery, dissipation, vicious habits, solitary vice, excessive venereal indulgence, lustful excesses, indolence, sloth, envy, jealousy, and anger (Forbes, Tweedie, and Conolly, 1849). By way of plethora, each of these factors could plausibly be seen as causing diseases. Suppose one is interested in discouraging some patient (e.g., a young aristocratic blood) from engaging in some practice (e.g., solitary vice). An obvious strategy is to represent that practice as liable to bring on some sickness or unhealthy state (blindness, perhaps). In short, one may describe the practice as more or less *sufficient* for bad health. However, since most people who engage in that practice do not actually become sick, the practice itself cannot really be *sufficient* for sickness. Moreover, since many people become sick without engaging in that practice, the practice isn't really *necessary* either. An obvious and natural solution is to portray the practice as one part of a complex cause that, *as a whole,* can be sufficient for sickness. One can then explain the good health of those who engage in the practice on the grounds that they happen to lack other essential elements in the complex sufficient cause, and one can explain the sickness of those who do not engage in the practice on the grounds that they succumbed to some other combination of factors that, while lacking the practice in question, was also sufficient for sickness. This is almost certainly the thinking behind common admonitions like "Don't go outside without a coat, you will catch cold."

Thus, it is reasonable to expect that persons who are eager to avoid certain practices will advance causal claims of this kind, and, conversely, that persons who advance such causal claims may ultimately be engaged in discouraging certain practices. In making such claims, the possible *effect* is usually less important to the person advancing the warning than avoiding what is assumed to be the *cause*. It is not surprising, for example, that in the Babylonian Talmud, whose authors were supremely eager to discourage violations of the religious law, causal claims of this form dominate discussion of disease and death (Carter, 1991). Given that almost all of the causal claims of early nineteenth-century physicians were also of this form, and that many of these claims explicitly identified the violation of moral or social norms as causes, we must begin to see the medicine of that period as an elaborate system among whose primary goals was reinforcing norms.

Of course, other factors contributed to the exclusive interest in this sort of cause. It is, after all, relatively difficult to find universal necessary causes of the kind that, today, dominate medical thinking—finding such causes is not a simple matter like finding shells on a beach. By contrast, it is easy to identify more or less plausible associations between diseases and such factors as, say, gluttony or indolence, and the associations become especially plausible given the intermediate link of plethora to which so many deviations seemed to contribute. No wonder that these associations seem to have been the basis for virtually all of earlier causal thinking in medicine.

In chapter 2, we saw that the use of bloodletting, the most prominent therapeutic measure of the early nineteenth century, was determined by the patient's behavior in relation to social and moral norms. Our investigation of the causal thinking in the period now reveals a similar connection. Regardless of whether practitioners were conscious of or would have readily agreed with this conclusion, we must see traditional medicine, chimbuki medicine, as an institution heavily, perhaps primarily, concerned with reinforcing social and moral norms. That seems to have been its function in society—if so, whatever benefits it may have generated were dependent on the discharge of that function. The nineteenth-century physician was concerned "that individuals were capable of playing their social roles successfully in a traditional structure of social position. Illness was for him an undue deviation from the norm" (Turner, 1967, p. 392).

David Wootton argues that the conceptual and technical requirements for the germ theory of disease were in place for decades, perhaps for as much as a century, before it was actually articulated, and he dates the beginning of doctors actually reducing disease from 1865, the year in which Joseph Lister adopted the practice of antiseptic surgery (Wootton, 2007). Why, he wonders, was good medicine delayed for so long? We can now see that, in spite of whatever overt goals may have been claimed by earlier physicians, what was called medicine in the early nineteenth century may actually have been about something entirely different. Exactly as we learned in our discussion of bloodletting, earlier causal talk was not wrong or irrational. Both were crucial parts of a reasonable, coherent, and remarkably tenacious system of thought and action that may have had enormous social utility (Rosenberg, 1979, pp. 1–5). And if the tenacity of this system cannot be explained by its success in achieving the eternal overt goals of medicine—the control or morbidity and the avoidance of death—one must look for a different kind of explanation. We thereby begin to see that earlier medical thinking and practice were profoundly different from our own and may have been driven by interests quite different from those that have dominated medicine since about the middle of the nineteenth century.

It should now be apparent how myopic, misleading, and just plain preposterous it is to judge traditional medicine simply on the basis of its capacity to increase longevity or to reduce general morbidity. These are certainly worthwhile goals, but who is to say that achieving them is more important or inherently valuable than other goals to which earlier medicine may have contributed? Admittedly, there is no way to measure the extent to which, if at all, traditional medicine actually fostered personal integrity, social cohesion, or psychological well-being, however, such potential benefits as these are certainly among those that must be appraised in deciding whether traditional medicine as a whole was or was not beneficial. And, of course, taking these as its goals should not be construed as minimizing the significance or social utility of chimbuki medicine. Whether in twentieth-century Zambia or in nineteenth-century Europe, the willful and widespread violation of norms can easily be more destructive to a society than is illness. So we must be cautious in claiming that all earlier medicine was *bad*—on the contrary, all things taken into account, chimbuki medicine may have served the interests of those who practiced it better than our medicine serves our interests today.

We turn now to another concept that, although frequently ignored, is important in understanding any medical system—the concept of a *quack*. We, today, have definite ideas about what quackery is, but every culture has had its own quacks, and the concept must always be understood as standing in opposition to the correlative idea of a regular practitioner. If, as I am arguing, in the course of the nineteenth century, traditional medicine—chimbuki medicine—gave way to our current system, we could expect there to have been a correlative shift in the concept of quackery. And, indeed, this concept did change significantly over the course of the nineteenth century. If properly understood, this change is another illustration of the contrast between chimbuki medicine and modern medicine and further evidence of the difference in the goals and expectations of the two systems.

4

The Early Nineteenth-Century Conception of Quackery

*That's the kind of fellow we call a [quack, one] advertising cures in
ways nobody knows anything about.*
—George Eliot, Middlemarch (1871–2)

*The proscription against advertising or unseemly publicity and the
rules for enlightened self-interest which govern the inevitable but
subtle competition between institutions or professionals are in the
"etiquette" category. There may be fragments of moral issues here,
but they are not mandatory obligations whose violation undermines
professional authenticity.*
—Edmund D. Pellegrino (1983)

Almost everywhere and almost always, quacks have been distinguished from regular medical practitioners. However, looking back
from our day, it is not entirely clear how quacks and regulars are to be
distinguished in earlier societies. Historians have commented on the
difficulty of drawing the distinction in a nontrivial way. For example,
in discussing medical practitioners in the sixteenth century, Margaret
Pelling and Charles Webster explain the problem as follows:

> The difficulties involved in framing consistent and historically
> fruitful criteria for isolating responsible medical practitioners from
> empirics and quacks have often not been fully appreciated. Terms
> such as *empiric* tend to be used without consistency or sound
> historical justification. Adoption of technical criteria for the isola-
> tion of empirics based on the legal code, professional attachments,
> or education attainment is practicable, but it tends to generate a
> trivial and unrealistically narrow conception of legitimate medical
> practice. Reference to more meaningful criteria related to profes-
> sional efficiency, reliability and responsibility, or the ideal of service
> rather than pecuniary gain, is difficult to operate because of lack of
> evidence. (Pelling and Webster, 1979, p. 166)

Historical discussions of quackery are usually anecdotal and, there-fore, more entertaining than enlightening (Porter, 1989); there have been few serious attempts to overcome the problem that Pelling and Webster have identified.

The root of the problem is easy to understand: central to our con-cept of quackery is the use of unproven medical practices. However, given that an interest in evidence-based medicine (i.e., an interest in determining which medical practices actually reduce morbidity) is a relatively recent phenomenon, applying our concept to earlier peri-ods or to non-Western medicine threatens to reduce everything to quackery—if there were *no* proven medical practices, from our point of view, *everything* must have been quackery. So, earlier on, how could the distinction have been made at all? In fact, our concept of quack-ery simply cannot be applied outside our own medical system, and understanding what other practitioners may have meant by quackery requires some understanding of the goals and purposes of medical practice—goals and purposes that cannot be assumed to have been the same as our own.

Regardless of how early nineteenth-century physicians may them-selves have characterized what they were doing, we have seen that, at the time, the goals of reducing mortality and morbidity were less prominent in medicine than the goal of reinforcing social and moral norms. From this alone, we might expect that earlier concepts of quackery would not focus, as our concept does today, on the use of practices whose effectiveness in reducing mortality and morbidity remain unproven. So how were quacks distinguished from regulars two hundred years ago?

I

In early nineteenth-century England, quackery was regarded as no less serious a problem than it is today—if anything it seems to have been more prevalent and to have attracted more medical attention. One writer judged that there were "more quacks in England than any-where else in the world" (Editor's Note, 1838–9a), and a British medical journal estimated that the ratio of quacks to regulars was about nine to one (Editor's Note, 1810). The British medical journal, *Lancet*, was founded, in part, to address the problem of quackery, and it quickly became the most widely distributed medical periodical in the world. Even in its first year, the editors claimed that *Lancet* was being read by more than ten thousand persons (Editor's Note, 1823), and twenty years later, the editors reported that "for upwards of the last eighteen years [*Lancet*] has commanded the largest circulation of any medical journal in the known world" (Editor's Note, 1843–4). Of course, readership was not limited to medical regulars: one writer observed that "every quack in England reads *Lancet* and takes especially good care to profit therefrom" (Pink and Blue, 1840–1, p. 322). In the early nineteenth century, *Lancet* and other contemporary British medical periodicals published hundreds of documents relating to quackery. These included general discussions, letters and editorials exposing and denouncing specific quacks, letters in which physicians defended themselves against charges of quackery, and even occasional letters in which self-acknowledged quacks tried to justify their own behavior. This literature provides an ample basis for an analysis of the prevailing concept of quackery—a concept that turns out to be significantly different from our own.

From an examination of this literature, four aspects of quackery emerge that warrant particular attention: first, as we would expect, the proven effectiveness of medical procedures was not central in identifying quackery; second, the commonest and most prominent charges brought against quacks were that they *advertised* and that they kept *secret* the contents of the remedies they prescribed; third, fully trained and duly licensed members of the profession—the so-called *regular* practitioners—frequently engaged in quackery; and finally, quackery among untrained or unlicensed practitioners was generally regarded as less significant than and, indeed, as a consequence of quackery among regulars. We will consider these four aspects one at a time.

(1) In the early nineteenth century, quacks seem often to have used precisely the same drugs and procedures that were used by orthodox physicians, and, for this reason, the proven effectiveness of medical practices was never an issue in the condemnation of quackery. The editors of medical periodicals, orthodox practitioners, and occasionally even self-confessed quacks all observed that the majority of quack nostrums were made from prescriptions formulated by famous and successful contemporary physicians. "Almost the whole of quack medicines are the revival of some once popular formula from our obsolete pharmacopoeias, or are the recipe of some well known medical man" (Editor's Note, 1838–9b). This observation is confirmed by the lists of ingredients in quack medicines that were occasionally published in *Lancet* and elsewhere; these medicines were invariably compounded from standard medical ingredients that were in common

use among orthodox physicians. Thus, early nineteenth-century physicians seem not to have been surprised that quack medicines sometimes seemed more effective than standard items in the pharmacopoeia. One regular physician, in complaining about the financial success of a nearby quack, admitted that several members of his own family had been treated by the quack and that the quack had, in fact, saved the life of his own father (Henderson, 1828–9). Another writer suggested that quacks could serve usefully in areas where there were insufficient regulars (Editor's Note, 1839–40). In the 1830s and early 1840s, several physicians proposed that quack medicines be systematically examined to determine whether or not they worked; those that were found to be genuinely effective were to be purchased from their creators and added to the standard pharmacopoeia (Editor's Review, 1829–30). The idea to test medicinal substances may or may not have been original at this time. In any case, the suggestion vividly reveals the inapplicability of our current concept—namely the use of unproven medications and procedures—as a basis for deciding which earlier practitioners were quacks. The problem with quackery was not that it involved the use of practices that were deemed ineffective; so what was the problem?

(2) Occasionally quacks were criticized for being inadequately knowledgeable about the use of their own remedies. In his *Dictionary*, published near the end of the eighteenth century, Samuel Johnson defined *quack* as "a boastful pretender to arts which he does not understand" (McAdam and Milne, 1965, p. 323). This definition reflects one possible etymology of *quack*: the word *quacksalver*, from whence we have *quack*, may have come into English from the Middle Dutch *quacsalver*, which may have been a corruption of *quicsilver*, Middle Dutch for mercury—among the strongest medications in the nineteenth-century pharmacopeia. *Webster's Third New International Dictionary* gives this etymology and suggests that the term acquired a pejorative sense from the use of mercury by persons who themselves lacked the understanding to treat effectively. Of course, none of this implies that the methods of the quack were ineffective; the objection is only that the quack himself did not understand his own methods or how to use his medications appropriately.

However, the most common basis for the charge of quackery was not simply a lack of understanding. In 1840, *Lancet* published an anonymous letter from a practitioner who identified himself as a member of the Royal College of Surgeons, a licentiate of the

Apothecaries Company, and yet a quack. (He signed his letter "Pink Saucer and Blue Light," in reference to an earlier letter objecting to his use of flamboyant means to attract customers.) (Pink and Blue, 1840–1). He observed, "Every chemist and druggist is to all intents and purposes a quack. They have all of them nostrums of their own. 'Bilious pills,' 'family pills,' 'dinner pills,' 'friends to females,' 'corn comforters,' etc." He described a fellow "member of the College and licentiate of the Hall" who had secretly obtained a copy of one of Dr. John Elliotson's prescriptions for cough. On finding that the prescription was effective, he had made up several hundred pills and sent them throughout the country "with a flaming paragraph, to which all the 'testimonials' of [such noted quacks as] Morrison, Eady, Franks, Holloway, and Solomon, are mere foolery." This letter reveals the two considerations that appear most frequently in contemporary discussions of quackery: first, the use of secret remedies, and second, the use of advertising and especially of testimonials. As a character in George Eliot's *Middlemarch* remarks, "That's the kind of fellow we call a [quack, one] advertising cures in ways nobody knows anything about" (Eliot, 1984, p. 494).

Editors of medical periodicals frequently denounced the use of secret remedies. Physicians who were fully trained and licensed and otherwise completely orthodox were regularly accused of quackery if they used remedies with secret ingredients. Beginning in 1835, Roderick Macleod, who had been licensed by the London College of Physicians and was a staff physician at St. George's hospital, was denounced for quackery through several issues of *Lancet* because he used secret remedies (Editor's Note, 1835–6). When the London Medico-Chirurgical Society closed its meetings to *Lancet* reporters, the editors retaliated by asking "this society [to] point out, the difference between the conduct of a quack, and that of a regular practitioner. Does not the first boast of the possession of a secret? Does not the regular practitioner boast of communicating his knowledge? . . . In its proceedings, therefore, does not the Medico-Chirurgical assume the character of a society of quacks?" (Editor's Note, 1829–30). The same aversion to secrecy led to the regular publication of lists of ingredients of the more popular quack medicines (Editor's Notes 1823). The purpose was to make quackery impossible by revealing the secrets on which it depended. *Lancet* even objected to exclusive practices in medical education and to the use of Latin or technical terminology; such practices were also seen as fostering a kind of secrecy and were, therefore, judged to be conducive to quackery (Editor's Note, 1835–6).

Quacks were also characterized by their use of advertising. Some writers felt that the term *quackery* could not be "extended to all advertised remedies [so long as] the component parts of a medicine are not publicly known, as well as the exact manner of preparing it" (Editor's Note, 1799). However, others objected to any form of advertising (Editor's Note, 1821). Sometimes even announcing a successful treatment or advertising a new medical text resulted in charges of quackery (M.D., 1845). One form of advertising was the use of testimonials, and even regular physicians were occasionally criticized for giving testimonials in favor of specific remedies (Cyclops, 1840–1). There were occasional letters in which medical societies such as the Royal College of Surgeons were urged to expel members who advertised or gave testimonials (A.Z., 1827). Physicians sometimes admitted to having given testimonials for quack medicines; in at least one case, a physician who admitted to have given testimonials and, therefore, to have practiced quackery argued that extenuating circumstances justified his behavior (Pink and Blue, 1840–1).

(3) It is fairly clear why orthodox practitioners objected to advertising and to the use of secret remedies: those who resorted to such measures gained an unfair advantage in the competition for patients. When one member of a medical faculty "advertised himself as an itinerant dentist," a local practitioner objected that this revealed "a monopolizing spirit" (Henderson, 1828–9, p. 614f). The editors of *Lancet* objected that "no individual belonging to [the medical profession] should be allowed to make a profit by any [secret] preparations beyond the limits of his own practice" (Editor's Note, 1838–9b). It is also clear why regular medical practitioners continued to resort to such practices even in the face of bitter denunciation by their peers and by the medical press: many physicians achieved only marginal financial success; many could not accumulate enough money in ordinary practice to provide for their basic needs. This drove them to exploit any advantage they could in receiving fees. One licensed physician, who admitted to practicing quackery, noted that if he were to stop, his "wife, children, and servants, would soon become more intimate with hunger and starvation than they have ever yet been." Thus, he concluded, while he respected the efforts to eradicate quackery, he respected himself more and he would, therefore, continue his

practice (Pink and Blue, 1840–1). Another physician admitted that he had given testimonials for quack medicines, but he observed that financial difficulties had driven him to do so and that he should not therefore be held culpable (Dendy, 1840–1).

As the preceding discussion illustrates, in the early nineteenth century, regular physicians could and often did engage in practices that were denounced as quackery. Regardless of how qualified a given practitioner was or how effective his treatments may have been, if he used secret medicines and advertised, he exposed himself to charges of quackery. These ideas are all clear in Thomas Percival's *Medical Ethics,* published in 1803, and widely used, throughout the remainder of the century, as a basis for ethical codes for the medical profession (Leake, 1927). Percival recommended that physicians discourage their patients from using quack medicines, but acknowledged that, because advertising is sometimes so effective, patients may become "obstinately bent on having recourse" to them (Leake, 1927, p. 103). He observed that effective preparations from the standard pharmacopoeia "ought not to be prescribed as quack medicines." He then observed that "no physician or surgeon should dispense a secret *nostrum,* whether it be his invention, or exclusive property." If such a preparation was really effective, doing so was "inconsistent with beneficence and professional liberality"; otherwise its use may imply "fraudulent avarice" (Leake, 1927, p. 104). Here we see all the elements that we have identified in other nineteenth-century criticisms of quackery—Percival presupposes that quack medicines are advertised and that their ingredients are kept secret. He admits that these medicines may be effective and are sometimes used by regular practitioners; however, he objects to their use on the grounds that, by using them, the practitioner gains an unfair advantage over their peers.

Because regular physicians sometimes practiced quackery, it was common to distinguish between regular and irregular quackery (Editor's Notes, 1840–1). The first was quackery by regularly trained and licensed physicians; irregular quackery was quackery by other persons—by the quasi-medical fringe. Particularly in *Lancet,* a surprisingly high percentage of published reports concerned the former.

(4) In the early nineteenth century, quackery within the medical profession was generally deemed a more serious problem than quackery in the quasi-medical fringe. There seem to have been several reasons for this. One regular practitioner, who himself

admitted to the practice of quackery, observed that the greatest quacks are "the very men who ought as the phrase goes, 'to uphold the honor and dignity of the profession'" (Pink and Blue, 1840–1, p. 323). In addition to practicing quackery directly, regular practitioners provided credibility for quack medicines by giving or selling endorsements and testimonials. The general opinion was that without endorsements from regular physicians, quack medicines would not have wide appeal and would cease to be a significant problem (Editor's Notes, 1846). By their own participation, and by endorsing quack medicines, regular practitioners contributed decisively to the practice of quackery. "Quackery is of itself weak and could not exist in its present rampant state if all the overt and covert assistance it obtains from medical men and medical names were entirely withdrawn" (Editor's Note, 1846).

But many writers saw an even more fundamental connection between quackery and orthodox medicine. As we have seen, most quack nostrum had been derived from prescriptions formulated by orthodox physicians. Several writers concluded that all quackery ultimately depended on orthodox medical knowledge and practice. But orthodox medicine included institutions and customs that seemed to promote secrecy. The editors of *Lancet* believed that the organization of medical colleges and companies, exclusive practices in medical education, and even the use of Latin and technical terminology created objectionable patterns of medical secrecy. The editors observed that the public was unable to distinguish between the secrecy of quacks and the secrecy of regulars who prescribed in Latin (Editor's Note, 1835–6). This orthodox and institutionalized secrecy seemed to provide the model for the secrecy that characterized quackery. With this in mind, the editors of *Lancet* reprinted, with their approval, an essay in which Adam Smith argued that the granting of medical degrees was the real source and essence of all forms of quackery (Editor's Note, 1840–1).

Quackery was, therefore, portrayed as a natural and almost inevitable outgrowth of institutionalized medicine. If so, it might be impossible to eliminate quackery until institutionalized medicine was purged of the practices that seemed to foster quackery. This explains, in part, why regular quackery was regarded as more insidious than irregular quackery, and why *Lancet's* first priority seems to have been reforming orthodox medicine and thereby eradicating regular quackery.

II

Certainly our concept of quackery has some areas of commonality with the early nineteenth-century concept. However, the preceding discussion shows that there are significant differences. Earlier practitioners may sometimes have associated the use of ineffective medical practices with quackery, but usually this was not a central concern. Usually, quacks were practitioners (whatever their training and however effective their treatments) who resorted to unfair strategies to gain patients. Of course, regular physicians, today, may still object to advertising and to other inappropriate attempts to attract patients. However, while the use of such practices might now be criticized as a violation of professional ethics or etiquette, it does not, by itself, warrant a charge of quackery. "In our times, the proscription against advertising or unseemly publicity and the rules for enlightened self-interest which govern the inevitable but subtle competition between institutions or professionals are in the 'etiquette' category. There may be fragments of moral issues here, but they are not mandatory obligations whose violation undermines professional authenticity" (Pellegrino, 1983, p. 195).

One can imagine that several factors contributed to the change in the concept of quackery. First, the earlier concept clearly reflected economic competition among practitioners; as the economic conditions of the profession improved, this dimension of the concept of quackery ceased to be a major concern. Second, during the course of the century, the efficacy of treatment became progressively more prominent as a criterion for appraising the success of medical treatment. Thus, the distinction between effective and ineffective medical procedures became progressively more important in distinguishing quacks from regulars. These two factors certainly influenced the changes that we have identified in the concept of quackery.

However, there is a third factor which, while more subtle, may be yet more fundamental than either of these, and, after the discussions in chapters 2 and 3, it may be apparent what this third factor will be. Suppose, as I have argued in earlier chapters, that nineteenth-century medicine was an institution whose primary objective was reinforcing social and moral norms. This would help explain strongly the *moral* concept of quackery in the earlier period. If one regards deviations from social and moral norms as significant causes of disease, and if physicians are expected to control disease through the inculcation of those norms, the use of unethical strategies to attract patients can be seen as a cynical repudiation of the very foundations of the medical system that the practitioner purports to apply. Thus, quackery, especially among regulars, was described as hypocrisy and even compared to heresy and to religious apostasy (Editor's Note, 1802, 1824, 1845).

In the middle of the nineteenth century, etiological investigations provided new concepts of disease that were no longer essentially linked to the violation of moral norms. With these concepts came new ways of thinking about medical practice. As we will see, old remedies were abandoned, not so much because they had been proven ineffective, as because they were incompatible with medicine's new, amoral role. With this change in the nature and role of medicine came changes in the concept of a regular medical practitioner and in the correlative concept of a quack. Thus, while changes in the concept of quackery may reflect changes in the economic status of the profession and in the effectiveness of available medical procedures, they may also be yet another superficial manifestation of very broad and fundamental changes in the role of medicine as social institution.

Decades ago, Erwin Ackerknecht warned us that "a fundamentally rational therapeutic method may be misunderstood because of its magic, semantic cloak" (Ackerknecht, 1946, p. 474). The reverse misunderstanding is also possible: what appears to be an essentially scientific vocabulary may cloak medical beliefs, concepts, and objectives totally alien from those that dominate our own thinking. In the early nineteenth century, physicians spoke so much as we now speak that we see continuity where, in fact, there was fracture, and we overlook strands of language that bind the practitioners of that period inextricably to other systems of thought. Arturo Castiglioni described early nineteenth-century physicians as scientists (Castiglioni, 1947, p. 760), and Michel Foucault celebrated the rise of pathological anatomy as the origin of a science of the individual (Foucault, 1973, p. 197). In fact, scientific medicine is a more recent development that began with the rise of a research agenda focusing on causes of disease (Carter, 2003). As we might expect from what we learned in chapter 3, one superficial clue that marks the origin of this new agenda is a change in talk about causes of diseases. As we now see, another such clue is a change in the professional expectations and standards of physicians.

Our next question must be how chimbuki medicine—an entirely reasonable, internally coherent, and remarkably tenacious system of thought and action, a system that may have had enormous social utility and that lasted for millennia—could possibly have collapsed within the space of a single generation. The key to understanding that collapse is discovering why, without significant argument or debate, bloodletting, the central therapy in chimbuki medicine, was suddenly abandoned without contemporary physicians even being aware that it was happening. We must now ask why physicians stopped therapeutic bloodletting.

5

The Edinburgh Bloodletting Controversy

Singular to say, the discussion [of the merits of bloodletting] . . .
instead of preceding, has followed the change, inasmuch as those who
are now contending for the advantages of bloodletting and antiphlo-
gistics in inflammation, are the very parties who acknowledge that
they no longer employ them.
—*John Hughes Bennett (1856–7b)*

In the early 1850s, William Pultney Alison, professor of the Practice of Physic at the University of Edinburgh, was nearing the end of an illustrious medical career. In three reflective clinical lectures, Alison considered whether it could really be, as contemporary medical theory allowed, that morbid inflammation arises because of "nearly opposite forms of constitutional disorder, and may therefore be fatal in very different ways?" (Alison, 1852, p. 493). In particular, could it be that the cellular effusions characteristic of pneumonia can be provoked either by "increased or deficient supply of blood" and are, therefore, "benefited in some cases by depleting [bloodletting], and in others by stimulating remedies?" If so, he inferred, for reasons about which "we must profess our entire ignorance," contrasting forms of pneumonia could dominate different historical periods. As an example, Alison observed that violent febrile pneumonia, which had frequently been encountered at the beginning of the century and which required massive abstractions of blood, seemed to have given way, by the 1850s, to a milder "typhoid form" of the disease that required supportive treatment but no bloodletting.

While discussing eleven cases of "well-marked pleurisy and pneumonia" then in his clinic, Alison observed, "I am strongly inclined to believe, from reflection on many other cases as well as these, that there has been a gradual change in the usual form and character of those inflammations, as occurring in the inhabitants of this country—and

73

that . . . they do not, in general, present the same intensity of local symptoms, nor the same amount of febrile reaction, as used to attend similar diseased actions . . . and therefore, that they do not furnish the same indications for bloodletting" (Alison, 1850, p. 164).

Alison reported having consulted with other experienced practitioners and having been assured that their observations were the same as his. Thus, pneumonia seemed to have become less intense and less often fatal and to require less energetic treatment.

John Hughes Bennett was twenty years younger than Alison and had been his student; he had also studied pathology in Paris. In the early 1850s, he was becoming established as a prominent clinician and pathologist in Edinburgh. In 1855, three years after the last of Alison's discussions, Bennett delivered a lecture entitled "The Present State of the Theory and Practice of Medicine." In one of several examples of current medical thought and practice, Bennett observed that pneumonia was now known always to require treatment "directly opposed" to bloodletting. It was for this reason, he concluded, that mortality from pneumonia had diminished since large bleedings had been abandoned, "and not because, as has been suggested by an eminent authority, inflammations, like fevers, have changed their types since the days of Cullen and Gregory" (Bennett, 1855, p. 19). In Bennett's published lecture, a footnote at the end of this sentence refers the reader to Alison's 1852 discussion.

By the time Bennett's lecture was published, Alison had retired from his professorship, but he immediately challenged Bennett's interpretation; Bennett responded, and other physicians were soon drawn into the dispute. The first phase of the ensuing debate is called the Edinburgh Bloodletting Controversy because the participants were associated with the University of Edinburgh and the discussions took place in meetings of the Medico-Chirurgical Society of Edinburgh. This *acute* phase of the controversy, which lasted for about one year, was characterized by heated verbal exchanges and politely worded insults. The debates touched on many issues, but one central question was why bloodletting had been almost completely given up over the preceding half century (an issue slightly different from the one about which Bennett and Alison initially disagreed). One disputant gave this concise account of the opposing views: according to Bennett, "The change in practice has been owing to an improved acquaintance with the pathology of diseases, rendering it apparent that bleeding never was the proper remedy for fevers and inflammations." By contrast, according to Alison, "A change has arisen by degrees in the constitution of such diseases, rendering the loss of blood, though formerly useful, an inadmissible treatment in the present day" (Christison, 1857–8, p. 577). Thus, in the debate, Alison *assumed* what he had earlier only conjectured, namely, that inflammation could be provoked in different ways and require opposite forms of treatment; he now used this conjecture to explain why bloodletting had been abandoned.

In the fall of 1857, the controversy entered a second *chronic* phase that carried it beyond Edinburgh: in a long essay, William O. Markham, a prominent London physician, agreed with Bennett that bloodletting had declined because of improvements in pathology and diagnosis, and he ridiculed the idea that pneumonia had changed in type. However, against Bennett (and with Alison) he argued that "bleeding is still a right remedy, highly to be respected, and of great service when rightly effected, and that it is nowadays less frequently used than needed" (Markham, 1857, p. 441). By this time, Alison and most of his original supporters had silently withdrawn from the contest, but for another ten years, Bennett and Markham, each supported by several other contributors, continued to debate the merits of taking blood and the reasons for the decline of the practice. By the end of the 1860s, the dispute gradually faded away without either party conceding defeat, but reverberations continued through the following decade.

Including both the acute and chronic phases, at least forty disputants contributed to the bloodletting controversy by publishing letters, essays, or books, or by participating in discussions that were transcribed and published. The debate had ramifications in America and in France, and the total literary remains fill hundreds of pages. The controversy has attracted the attention of twentieth-century historians (Carter, 2010, p. 2).

The bloodletting controversy is a curious episode: everyone agreed, from the outset, that bloodletting, which had been a standard therapy in Western medicine for more than two millennia, had been all but given up and that this had happened silently, almost without discussion or debate. This profound change seemed no less remarkable to those who experienced it than it does to us today. "Singular to say," Bennett observed, "the discussion [of the merits of bloodletting] . . . instead of preceding, has followed the change, inasmuch as those who are now contending for the advantages of bloodletting and antiphlogistics in inflammation, are the very parties who acknowledge that they no longer employ them" (Bennett, 1856–7b, p. 1000). For our purposes, the bloodletting controversy is important because it provided a forum in which those who had experienced the change in therapeutics could express their opinions about what had taken place and why. Thus, the controversy sheds light on the decline of bloodletting and on the eventual collapse of chimbuki medicine.

One early disputant observed that "every sane man but Dr. Bennett" agrees with Alison, and that Bennett stands entirely alone in his views on this subject (Alison, 1856–7b, p. 1050). Indeed, while Bennett claimed to have received letters of support, in the first phase of the controversy (until Markham entered the debate in 1857), only one participant published anything supporting Bennett (Carter, 2010, p. 3). By contrast, twentieth-century writers, who are more likely to dismiss the whole practice of bloodletting as a monumental lapse of rationality, have generally preferred Bennett's views to Alison's. Lester S. King described Bennett as a fellow traveler on "the modern highroad of progress" while dismissing Alison as "a True Believer" in things past—a kind of intellectual dinosaur (King, 1961, p. 12f). But given what we know about the extensive social and moral ramifications of bloodletting, one must question the idea that strictly rational considerations, such as those Bennett proposed to explain the decline of bloodletting, could, within a single generation, have overthrown a practice as ancient, as widespread, and as deeply entrenched as bloodletting; something more must have been involved.

In this chapter, I will support a version of Alison's account of the change in therapy: I will argue that one reasonable interpretation of the doctrine of a change of type partly explains the decline of bloodletting. In chapter 6, we will see that, speaking very loosely, Bennett may also have been partly correct in thinking that "an improved acquaintance with the pathology of diseases" contributed to the decline of bloodletting, but this did not happen in the way that Bennett seems to have believed.

I

Alison, who was certainly the most subtle and profound of the many participants in the controversy, explicitly allowed that the rise of modern pathology *contributed* to the decline of bloodletting, but he denied that the change in therapy could "be explained merely in this way" (Alison, 1855–6, p. 784). By contrast, neither Bennett nor any of Alison's original supporters seems to have entertained the idea that bloodletting declined because of a combination of different factors.

In particular, aside from Alison, none of the original disputants seems to have allowed that "an improved acquaintance with the pathology of diseases" *and* changes in the total disease picture could *both* have worked against the popularity of bloodletting. Yet, obviously, these explanations are not mutually exclusive. At least three times, before the bloodletting controversy began, both factors had been mentioned *together* in explaining the change in therapy, and some later writers assumed, without question, that considerations of both kinds influenced the decline of venesection (Carter, 2010, p. 3). Changing scientific opinions did undermine support for bloodletting, although, as we will see, for the most part, these changes came *after* the use of bloodletting had seriously declined, and the changes were not of the sort that one might have expected.

So what did Alison believe about the change of type? According to Alison, the doctrine of change of type was "that all causes, capable of exciting diseased action in the animal economy, or more probably, that the liability to diseased actions in the different departments of the animal economy itself, are subject to variations" (Alison, 1855–6, p. 772f). Thus, in brief, either the causes of a given disease or the vulnerability to disease (or both) may change. Given this account, the doctrine is a disjunction of two possibilities of which Alison preferred the second (altered liability). However, the disjuncts are not mutually exclusive; Alison never rejected the first possibility (changing causes), and most of what he wrote could apply given either way of thinking. We will focus on the second disjunct (altered liability), but it is worth noting that a few texts support the first: Alison allowed that the intensity of disease could reflect unknown atmospheric changes (Alison, 1850, p. 165). Moreover, other disputants, less cautious than Alison, compared changes in the intensity of pneumonia to changes in the virulence of eruptive fevers like smallpox; it seemed plausible that variations in smallpox mortality reflected changes in the causes of the disease rather than in the vulnerability of victims, and this suggested that inflammations like pneumonia could also change (Carter, 2010, p. 4).

In spite of these passages, Alison and his followers seem usually to have regarded change of type as a theory about the human constitution—about human vulnerability to disease. In what was to become a famous and frequently quoted passage in the controversy, Thomas Watson wrote that "the human constitution is [capable,] from influences to us unknown, of undergoing alterations, in respect to the manner in which it is affected by inflammation, and by the reputed remedies of inflammation. For my own part, I am firmly persuaded, by my own observation, and by the records of medicine, that there are waves of time through which the sthenic and the asthenic characters of disease prevail in succession, and that we are at present living amid one of its adynamic phases" (Watson, 1856–7, p. 1088). J.A. Easton, another of Alison's supporters, wrote that "while maintaining that the inflammation of today, is the same in character and essence as the inflammation of a thousand years ago, it does not follow that . . . mankind, in all ages, should be similarly affected by its power" (Easton, 1857–8, p. 709). Yet another supporter explained change of type as "a change in the bodily constitution of the community, [possibly] caused by a change in the kind of food [that was available]" (Christison, 1857–8, p. 579). Finally, W.O. Markham explained change of type as the idea that "the human constitution has been so influenced by the external conditions to which it has been of late years subjected, as to have undergone some decided modification—such as would be visible, for instance, in the effects of disease upon the body" (Markham, 1857, p. 493).

Change of type was never carefully explained, but a few of Alison's comments are enlightening: he admitted that changes in human liability "are made known to us only by the variation of [disease] phenomena themselves" (Alison, 1855–6, p. 788). He also wrote that changes in type are "ultimate facts, to be carefully observed, arranged, and classified, but which we are not to expect to be resolved into any others [simpler and better understood]" (Alison, 1855–6, p. 788).

Bennett found it easy to attack this vague doctrine. After listing the pathological changes characteristic of inflammation, he asked, "How can it be shown that any of these necessary changes have of late years undergone any modification? If a healthy man receive a blow, or any other injury is inflicted on his person, are the resulting phenomena in these days in any way different from those which took place in the days of Cullen and Gregory? . . . This has not yet been shown" (Bennett, 1856–7a, p. 773). "Is one to believe," he continued, "that the whole people of this country, since the days of Cullen and Gregory, have become so debilitated—that their constitutions have become so altered for the worse, that attacked by the same lesion, and to the same extent, there is no longer the same reaction . . .. Are our soldiers and sailors, workmen or others, physically less capable of exertion than formerly?" (Bennett, 1856–7a, p. 775). "For my own part," Bennett continued, "I have earnestly sought for, but cannot discover, a shadow of evidence for such a belief." Moreover, if the doctrine was intended to explain the decline of bloodletting, similar changes must have been happening all over the world since, by the 1850s, Indian physicians were also bleeding their patients less frequently than they once had done. Bennett asked, "Is it not more reasonable then to think, that the alteration of the practice in India results from a change in precept and example, and that the continuance of the practice in Italy and in the wards of M. Bouillaud [in France], is owing to the absence of such change, rather than to suppose that inflammation alters in type, just where the practice alters, but remains stationary in those countries, and even in those wards of an hospital, where it does not?" (Bennett, 1856–7a, p. 776).

Alison had no effective response to these criticisms: he accepted Bennett's claim that no change could be demonstrated "in the essential *nature* of inflammations," but insisted that there could still have been changes "in their usual *symptoms*, local and general, which had been followed by a suitable change in treatment" (Alison, 1856–7a, p. 857). Alison expressed incredulity at the idea that everyone since Hippocrates had simply been wrong about the utility of medicine's most cherished therapy (Alison, Reply 1856–7b, p. 976). He insisted that he personally had observed the change in type over the course of his career (Alison, 1855–6). Finally, he quoted letters from colleagues who reported having noticed changes of the same kind.

Notwithstanding this spirited and emotional defense, support for change in type soon declined. By 1864, Watson conceded that the doctrine may be false, and by the late 1860s, it seems to have been generally believed that Bennett and Markham had conclusively refuted the doctrine (Carter, 2010, p. 5).

However, by itself, the idea of a change in type seems relatively innocuous: it seems quite reasonable that variations in the human constitution—variations resulting from changes in diet, for example—can affect vulnerability to diseases including inflammation and pneumonia. Indeed, it is precisely changes of these kinds to which Thomas McKeowen has attributed the striking change in mortality that resulted in the long-term doubling of life expectancy in England between 1680 and 1942 (and, at the very heart of this interval, of course, is the very period we are considering). "We are in the profoundly unsatisfactory situation of not having anything resembling an adequate understanding of the most important single event in modern history, the revolution in life expectancy. McKeowen thought he knew the answer. He

79

argued that the major factor was better resistance to disease, and that the only thing that could have made this possible was better nutrition. His argument has come under repeated and sustained attack, but it remains the best explanation we have" (Wootton, 2007, p. 276). And even Bennett admitted that the doctrine could conceivably be true (Bennett, 1856–7c, p. 1090).

So why has change of type been consistently rejected? There are at least two reasons (but we will not consider the second until the penultimate section of this chapter): For one thing, however plausible the doctrine may be *in itself*, change of type seems problematic when used to account for the decline of bloodletting. If one begins by believing (with Bennett and with most twentieth-century writers) that bloodletting was ultimately only a big mistake, it follows that any explanation of its decline *that implicitly justifies its earlier use* must also be wrong. Holding that, because there has been a change of type, bloodletting is no longer justified seems to imply that before the change, bloodletting may have been justified, so, from the point of view of anyone who categorically rejects bloodletting, it must follow that this explanation for the decline of bloodletting is incorrect. Thus, while this never became fully explicit in the debate, the logic of the argument forced Alison and his camp to provide a plausible justification for bloodletting in general. But providing such a justification was difficult given the belief, on which Bennett repeatedly insisted, that bloodletting could only be beneficial if it modified the morbid changes that constitute inflammation. Alison admitted that bloodletting could not modify the disease process once it began, but held out for the possibility that it may influence the patient *before* observable morbidity actually set in—this was why, as everyone had always maintained, bloodletting was only effective if used at the very outset of disease (Alison, 1855–6, p. 772). Bennett had no trouble disposing of this weak response and, from a logical point of view, that ended the debate. By specifying the conditions under which alone bloodletting could be deemed justified, Bennett had, in effect, defined the terms of the dispute in such a way that Alison's position became indefensible. However, it is simplistic to think (as Bennett insisted) that bloodletting could be useful in only one way (just as it is simplistic to think that only one cause led physicians to give it up). And, since my goal in this chapter is merely to defend one version of Alison's doctrine (not to give a comprehensive account of bloodletting or to explain completely its decline), we are not limited by Bennett's way of defining the terms of dispute.

We have seen that bloodletting was at the center of medical interests in defining and reinforcing social norms. Given this understanding of how bloodletting functioned in nineteenth-century medicine, it will be easier to understand how the practice quickly lost much of its appeal. I will argue that, given existing beliefs about bleeding, widely shared opinions of contemporary demographic and social changes (whether true or imaginary) implied that bloodletting should be drastically reduced. Thus, quite apart from Bennett's improvements in pathology and diagnosis (which, I repeat, may certainly have helped undermine belief in bloodletting), physicians may, indeed, have stopped bleeding partly because of what could reasonably be described as a change in type.

II

In the middle of the nineteenth century, physicians believed they had witnessed the emergence of a new mode of life—life as a working-class city dweller. "In the commencement of the century, the agricultural or outdoor workers formed three-fourths or more of the inhabitants; now [1857], the indoor or town and manufacturing population far outnumber the former" (Turnbull, 1857–8, p. 187). Physicians believed that this demographic change had important consequences for the human constitution and for medicine.

Physicians joked, grimly, that not a healthy person could be found in the whole of London, and the main reason seemed to be that city dwellers experienced "an unusual excitement of the whole system" (Abernethy, 1824, p. 6). In the large cities, "most things are in the extreme, and life is an intellectual or physical fever—a state of excitement or collapse" (Armstrong, 1825, p. 262). London physicians regularly treated "patients whose constitutions have suffered from indulgences in all the vices, and from all the nicest excitement to which man is exposed amid this vast concourse of human beings" (Wardrop, 1833, p. 236). Thus, city life was believed typically to involve intense mental and emotional excitement and irritability. But the dangers of extreme excitement were compounded by overconsumption—especially by the abuse of alcohol. This became a problem because working city dwellers generally had more disposable income than their rural counterparts.

> A large proportion of the individuals employed in various working departments obtain high wages, which they spend chiefly in direct sensual gratification of the grossest kind. It is no uncommon circumstance for men employed in the coal business, brewers' servants,

draymen, porters, and others, who are, generally speaking, fine robust men coming out of the country, to consume 6, 8, 10 and 12 pots of porter a day, besides gin, and a full allowance of animal food. You certainly see many of these who, if you regard fullness of flesh and ruddiness of complexion as signs of health, may be considered as fine specimens. But these persons are subject to inflammatory attacks of the most violent kind, which they bear very ill. (Lawrence, 1825, p. 406)

One London physician wrote that excessive consumption "lays the foundation of by far the greater portion of human maladies" (Barlow, 1849a, p. 751). We have noted that etiological discussions frequently included such terms as "excessive diet," "gross and luxurious diet," "gluttony," "high feeding," and "full and stimulating diet." Overconsumption of alcohol was listed as a possible cause of virtually every recognized disease (Forbes, Tweedie, and Conolly, 1849).

Among the inhabitants of large towns, many people satisfied traditional criteria for bleeding: in town "all kinds of luxurious indulgences which tend to repletion are carried to the utmost extent. We know that sedentary habits, which favor such repletion, are very prevalent, and, therefore, all the habits and circumstances calculated to produce *direct* plethora—that state in which high inflammatory action will occur, and in which that inflammatory action will require the most active means" (Lawrence, 1829–30, p. 271). But most city-dwelling patients—in particular, city dwellers of the lower orders—were different: they combined overindulgence (especially in alcohol) with intense mental excitement and physical exertion. This gave rise to a new category of patient, different from the ideal types in terms of which traditional therapies were defined, and it was unclear what form of medical treatment was appropriate. Some physicians argued that city dwellers required even more extensive abstractions of blood than rural patients, but most physicians reached the opposite conclusion (Clutterbuck, 1838a, p. 168). Among the factors traditionally recognized as rendering bloodletting, "unnecessary or hurtful" were "a constitution broken down by drinking, starvation, or excessive exercise of body or mind" (Cumming, 1853, p. 242)—almost exactly the conditions that seemed to characterize industrial workers. Thus, most physicians concluded that, if these people were to be bled at all, only small quantities of blood could be taken and this could only be done with extreme caution (Blundell, 1828). In town, "the constitution of

patients is broken by intemperance, or enfeebled by deteriorated air";
thus, in London, it was "seldom safe to take blood," whereas "in the
country, a different practice may be pursued" (Cooper, 1823, 1823–4).
One physician explained that among "a healthy, rural population," he
would "not hesitate to bleed largely," but "in large towns, with a demor-
alized, ill-fed, ill-housed, ill-clothed and drunken population, the large
abstraction of blood might certainly be hazardous" (Stephens, 1857–8).
"In large towns, and more particularly in hospitals [where physicians
encountered poor patients], bloodletting exercises an injurious effect
on the vast majority of the cases of pneumonia . . . while . . . in country
districts, . . . cases may be found in which a single bloodletting will
arrest the further progress of the disease" (Easton, 1857–8, p. 709).
The clear consensus was that working-class city dwellers should not
ordinarily be bled.

Alison and his supporters repeatedly insisted that one usually
encounters febrile inflammatory pneumonia (the form of pneumonia
that called for bloodletting) only among "persons of rank" who are
seen at home in private practice (Alison, 1855–6, p. 782f) or in rural
practices, where most patients still followed "a traditional and healthy
mode of life" (Easton, 1857–8, p. 709). In city hospitals, physicians
confronted only "persons of the lower ranks of life" who required
supportive treatment (Alison, 1850, p. 162). Alison observed, "I could
show more examples of inflammatory diseases . . . and of the effects
of bloodletting on them, . . . in one forenoon, by visits to dispensary
patients, than in a three months course of attendance on the clinical
wards of the infirmary" (Alison, 1855–6, p. 783). Thus, while bleeding
was still appropriate among wealthy city dwellers or in the country,
it was inadmissible among the lower-class working people ordinarily
seen in teaching hospitals.

For our purposes, it matters little whether these supposed changes in
population and lifestyle were real or imaginary—it is essential only that
physicians *believed* there had been important social changes and that,
because of these changes, bloodletting was less frequently indicated.
However, it is worth noting that these common beliefs may have had a
basis in fact. The first half of the nineteenth century witnessed unprec-
edented urban growth. Moreover, improving living standards among
the middle and lower classes created new markets both for commodi-
ties (including alcohol and spirits) and for services (including medical
care). These changes have been described as the birth of the consumer society (McKendrick, Brewer, and Plumb, 1982). A new kind of

medical professional—the general practitioner (Loudon, 1986)—provided medical care for most working-class city dwellers: "The great mass of the population in this kingdom is attended by general practitioners; such is the case in the army and navy, and with the middling and lower classes" (Lawrence, 1827, p. 633). So through the early nineteenth century, practitioners of a new kind cared for patients of a new class who did not conform to the categories in terms of which bloodletting was traditionally conceived. As these patients became more numerous and gained greater disposable wealth, treatment episodes involving general practitioners and working-class city dwellers became a new norm for medical care, and in these treatment episodes, bloodletting was judged to be inappropriate. It should now be clear that, from the point of view of contemporary physicians, city life did involve changes in "the liability to diseased actions in the different departments of the animal economy itself" (Alison, 1855–6, p. 788), that is, what Alison called a change of type. Moreover, given the nature of this change, bloodletting seemed inappropriate for those who constituted the largest (and an ever-expanding) class of patients. It was clear that there would be a drastic reduction in the use of bloodletting.

Watson thought in terms of "waves of time through which the sthenic and the asthenic characters of disease prevail in succession" (Watson, 1856–7, p. 1088), and some physicians looked forward to a time when "a reflux in the constitution of fever will present it again in its sthenic dress, and again make the lancet its remedy" (Christison, 1857–8, p. 595). But other physicians understood more clearly the nature of the change that was occurring. In supporting Alison against Bennett, W. Turnbull wrote:

> It is difficult to estimate properly the influence on the human frame of a town life—of an indoor existence—of a tea and coffee diet—of perambulators, and the traveling-made-easy rail—and of head-work instead of limb-work . . . .. If, then, the change of type in disease depend[s] upon a change in the habits and occupation of the people—upon an indoor life—upon crowding together in towns and villages—and upon the nervous system having too much work, and the muscular too little—I see no reason to expect a return of the sthenic diathesis; but, on the contrary, I should look for the tendency to be in the opposite direction, as all the causes I have glanced at must augment in force with the increase in number and density of the population, and with a greater and greater proportion

being employed in other than pastoral and agricultural pursuits. (Turnbull, 1857–8)

Thus, the effects of the change of type, far from being cyclical, "will be more and more marked in each succeeding generation." Turnbull saw that the change of type was irreversible and, therefore, that therapeutic bloodletting was doomed. Other observers reached similar conclusions (Editor's Review, 1954, p. 199).

III

In the fall of 1857, William O. Markham entered the bloodletting debate. Like Alison, Bennett, and Watson, Markham was a leading figure in contemporary British medicine. Over the next few years, he frequently lectured on bloodletting; several of his lectures were published or reported in *Lancet* or in the *British Medical Journal*, and they provoked numerous responses.

Markham frequently discussed the possibility of a change of type. He asked, "In the history of the world, is there anywhere recorded a state of society comparable to that amidst which we exist?" (Markham, 1857, p. 494). In modern society, he observed, "human beings have been . . . massed together, and subjected, in body and in mind, to new conditions of existence; and is it reasonable to believe that they remain unaffected and unchanged in their bodily and in their mental organizations? Most assuredly not. Need we, then, invoke any other explanation than this, to tell us why it is that large masses of the inhabitants of towns and cities bear large bleedings ill?" He pointed out that "the entire history of the mechanic's life, . . . is antagonistic to high health. His mind is more stretched and more excited—his body more worked and more stimulated, than the rustic's. One item alone in the long catalogue will readily suggest that some great change must inevitably be worked by it on his body: I mean the enormous amount of spirituous drinks annually consumed by him." These working city dwellers constitute "the class which finds its way into our public hospitals." And the members of this class are the persons who seemed to illustrate the change of type. Thus, "the argument in favor of a change of type is drawn from the results of practice as witnessed amongst enormous masses of human beings, who are subjected to deteriorating influences, in kind and in degree differing vastly from the influences surrounding men in former days." By contrast, "there is no evidence offered of any change in the type of diseases amongst the healthy agricultural population. On the contrary, bleeding . . . is still an ordinary daily remedy for inflammation occurring in that class." Markham also pointed out that military physicians continued profuse bloodletting and made no appeal to the doctrine of change of type.

However, Markham insisted the social changes he identified were adequate to explain the decline of bloodletting without resorting to "any imagined change in the type of disease," and he emphatically rejected change of type. Why was Markham unwilling to accept, as a true change of type, the very modifications of human nature that seemed to follow the social developments he himself stressed and that contemporary writers identified as the basis of the doctrine? As we saw earlier, one reason Bennett rejected change of type may have been that, by accepting the doctrine, he would have been forced to admit that bloodletting had once been appropriate. Markham rejected change of type for exactly the opposite reason: he ardently believed in bloodletting, and he regarded the doctrine of change of type as "the greatest obstacle" to its continued use: "if it could be satisfactorily shown that the theory [of change of type] was erroneous, then the profession would be bound to reconsider the whole matter, and would, I am satisfied, once again take the lancet in hand and bleed their patients" (Markham, 1866, pp. 437, 490). Markham felt that by accepting, as a true change of type, the modifications of human nature that followed irreversible contemporary social developments, one was forced, like Turnbull, to conclude that bloodletting was doomed. So, while admitting everything Turnbull (and possibly even Alison) required for a change of type, he rejected the doctrine.

However, this left Markham teetering on the brink of inconsistency. As we have seen, change of type was usually taken to mean that the human constitution can change in response to variations in factors like diet, alcohol consumption, or way of life. This was how most writers, including both Alison and Markham himself, explained the doctrine. Markham specifically admitted that these factors could change the human *constitution*: "remove the pale mechanic from the town, give him pure air, and let the rays of the heavens shine clearly on him, give him wholesome food and drink, *and you rapidly change the constitution of the man.*" Yet in the very next paragraph, when discussing and rejecting change of type, Markham writes, "The *constitution of man*, as far as we have any proof, is now what it has ever been" (Markham, 1857, p. 493). Markham saw that people were changed by city life, but he also wanted to support bloodletting, and he regarded change of type as an obstacle to that practice. The result was inconsistency.

Markham denied change in type while, at the same time, ascribing the decline of bloodletting to the very social changes that Turnbull and others identified as the basis of the doctrine *and* insisting that the general belief in change of type had become the greatest single obstacle to the practice of bloodletting. Since, as I pointed out above, it matters little whether the social changes physicians thought they had witnessed were real or imaginary, Markham's concessions amount to an endorsement of the very thesis for which I am here arguing: bloodletting declined (in part) because physicians believed that changes they observed in the human constitution made the practice inappropriate.

Bennett and Markham rejected change of type as an explanation for the decline of bloodletting in part because it implied *both* that bloodletting had once been appropriate (which Bennett, like some modern commentators, could not accept) *and* that it had become irreversibly inappropriate (which Markham could not accept). We will now consider a second reason why the doctrine has never seemed plausible as an explanation for the decline of bloodletting: Alison's account was hopelessly vague and ambiguous. Did the essence of disease somehow change, or were there changes in human vulnerability? Were the changes periodic in a way that meant bloodletting might again become appropriate, or were they unique and essentially irreversible? Was change of type an ultimate fact, or could it be explained in terms of changing diet or mode of life? Alison made no serious attempts to answer such questions. Moreover, he and his supporters gave inconsistent accounts of the theory, and Markham exploited these inconsistencies to discredit the doctrine. Alison seems to have realized the decline of bloodletting reflected something independent from (and perhaps more fundamental than) the simple growth of pathological knowledge, but he was unable to explain coherently what it was. Instead of recognizing that social class was one factor (among others) that affected the total disease picture and the selection of therapy, and that changes in class structure would, therefore, bring changes in prevailing therapies, Alison introduced, as "ultimate facts," undefined and untestable changes of type. The connection between evolving social classes and changing therapies was obscured by being presented in quasi-metaphysical categories.

Alison accused Bennett of assuming that change of type involved "the essential *nature* of inflammations," rather than a change in the manifestation of inflammation in the patient—a reasonable mistake given the equivocal way in which the doctrine had been presented. In part, this obscurity may have enabled Markham to pass off an inherently inconsistent position as though it were a telling criticism of the doctrine. The same obscurity clouds twentieth-century discussions of the decline of bloodletting. Peter H. Niebyl writes that the revolution in therapy "was influenced by social factors," and he concludes that "the cause and the success of the Bloodletting Revolution . . . can in large measure be found in the earlier demobilization of military surgeons" (Niebyl, 1977, p. 472). Thus, while ignoring demographic changes that may have been even more important to evolving medical practices, Niebyl was clearly sensitive to the impact of social changes on bloodletting. However, he (like Bennett) seems to have regarded change of type as about disease essences rather than about the human constitution, and he thereby missed the connection between change of type and social change. He writes: "The 'change of type' explanation seems antiquated because our definition of disease entities today is even more rigorous than that of the early contagionists" and "the changes in [medical] practice were simply too great and too extensive to be accounted for by local epidemics alone" (Niebyl, 1977, p. 481). Niebyl seems to assume that what Alison called change of type was really a sequence of local epidemics of different diseases that Alison (supposedly) failed to recognize as such because his views had "destroyed the specificity of disease." As a result, while Niebyl considers the impact of episodic crop failures and of large-scale unemployment on human susceptibility to disease, he never associates these factors with change of type. By contrast, one of Alison's supporters used precisely these two factors to explain and to illustrate how human liability could change and had changed, that is, how Alison's change of type had taken place (Christison, 1857–8, p. 581).

John Harley Warner is clear that there were two versions of the change-in-type theory: one focusing on changes in disease essences and "a second version" according to which, rather than diseases themselves, "the constitution of the human body had undergone a change" (Warner, 1980, p. 246). Citing Turnbull, he even associates this second version with "the destructive effects of urbanization." But, having shown that, through the early decades of the century, therapeutic changes followed epidemiological changes as typhus and relapsing fever (the former "clinically perceived to be asthenic, the later . . . clearly sthenic" [Warner, 1980, p. 243]) alternatively swept the British

Isles, Warner essentially ignores the second version of the theory and concludes only that "an examination of epidemiological changes and their therapeutic correlates during this period reveals that there was some existential basis for the change-of-type theory" (Warner, 1980, pp. 257, 247). Like Bennett, Markham, and Niebyl, Warner ends up thinking primarily in terms of the first version of the theory. He then concludes that "in large measure this theory was a product of the Edinburgh medical profession's status anxieties." However, suppose one adopts the second version of the theory—the one preferred by Alison. Then, given the role of social class in the selection of therapy, perceived demographic changes become a plausible experiential basis for a change of type.

As the advancing class of working city dwellers exploited progressively more of the available medical resources, ordinary physicians saw fewer and fewer persons belonging to the economic class within which bloodletting seemed most appropriate. As they themselves expressed it, physicians witnessed an irreversible change of type because of which bloodletting had become inappropriate. These are two descriptions for one and the same change. From whichever point of view one describes it, the decline of bloodletting was inevitable.

In 1857, Markham supported Bennett by rejecting the idea that the decline of bloodletting could have occurred simultaneously with the advance of medical knowledge and yet have been independent of that new knowledge. But surely it would have been even less credible to suppose that bloodletting could decline simultaneously with the emergence of working-class city dwellers (and, therefore, simultaneously with the reorganization of the social classes in terms of which bloodletting was traditionally conceived) and yet be independent of the rise of that new class. While no one would deny that the growth of medical science influenced therapy, social change—change of type—was at least as destructive of the traditional rationale for bloodletting as anything discovered in a pathology laboratory.

IV

We must now draw together the main strands of our story: as we have seen, according to early nineteenth-century physicians, bloodletting was required for patients whose behavior violated, or even threatened to violate, various social and moral norms. By taking blood, physicians worked a kind of blood atonement that compensated for and in some sense may even have justified those violations. While contemporary physicians would have seen and described this as healing their patients (and to some extent they were no doubt right), we must suspect that supporting those norms was the primary benefit—the *reason for being*—of the entire medical system. This possibility receives independent support from the particular concept of disease causation that was then in use and also from what was the contemporary concept of quackery. Because we can interpret early nineteenth-century medicine in this way, we refer to it as *chimbuki* medicine. But the use of this term should not suggest any disrespect either for the real chimbuki or for nineteenth-century physicians. Our use of the term should not be taken to imply that either system was ineffective or even that, taken as a whole, one or the other was less beneficial to society than our current system of medicine. The term is intended only to underscore the profound difference between these systems of medicine and our own and to help us keep clearly in mind what seems to have been the chief objective of earlier medicine—namely, insuring that patients lived lives in harmony with prevailing moral and social standards.

Then, over the space of a single generation, things changed profoundly. The physicians who witnessed this change described it as a change in "the liability to diseased actions in the different departments of the animal economy," something they referred to as a *change in type* (Alison, 1855–6, p. 772f). Judging by contemporary accounts, it may be possible to explain the change these physicians experienced in terms of a change in their clientele: physicians seem to have encountered fewer and fewer patients who were members of the classes in terms of which the use of bloodletting was traditionally explained and justified. Bloodletting seemed to have no place in treating their new patients, and its use declined precipitously. But since bloodletting was the central therapy in chimbuki medicine, with the decline of bloodletting, chimbuki medicine itself was in serious jeopardy.

It should now be clear why the decline in bloodletting, and indeed the collapse of the entire medical system of which bloodletting was a part, was not preceded or even accompanied by any discussion or debate. The changes in medical practice stemmed from *social* changes, that is, from changes that occurred within each physician's individual practice. In confronting a new patient, each physician selected a course of therapy depending on the patient's total circumstances (including the social class from which the patient came). Because of changes in the classes from which most patients were drawn, bloodletting was judged to be required in fewer and fewer cases. None of this required or motivated any discussion among practitioners. By contrast, suppose there had been some new discovery or some newly conceived argument that counted against bloodletting (suppose, in other words, that, at some point, bloodletting had actually been contested). Such a development would have provoked discussion and debate. But that never happened: there was, in fact, never any attempt to refute bloodletting. And that, of course, was because everyone knew that *it worked*—as Pierre-Charles-Alexandre Louis proved and as even John Bennett admitted, if administered properly, bloodletting was effective against fever and inflammation. Since the change in therapy all played out within the practices of individual physicians, at first no one could have been more than dimly aware that bloodletting was in *universal* decline. Ultimately, however, the declining use of bloodletting became obvious—William Alison wrote to his colleagues and confirmed that, in this respect, their experience was like his own. At that point, beginning in about 1850, there was discussion and debate about *why* bloodletting had been given up, but by then it was an accomplished fact, and there were never any arguments that it *should* be given up.

Of course, and this is extremely important, even as practitioners became aware that bloodletting was being abandoned, no one could have realized that their entire medical system was breaking up. Since there was, as yet, nothing with which to compare chimbuki medicine, the fact that the whole system was collapsing could only become apparent after a new system arose, that is, it could only become apparent in retrospect. Looking back, we can now see what happened and why; in the 1850s, even while it was underway, a change this fundamental would have been not only inapparent but literally inconceivable.

So far we have a partial account of the collapse of traditional medicine, but our account is far from complete. As we will see, beyond social changes, other factors also contributed to the decline of bloodletting. But these other factors can be appreciated only after we understand one absolutely crucial innovation in medical thought that, from a conceptual point of view, *both* entailed the final overthrow of chimbuki medicine *and* prepared the way for what was to follow. Thus, in addition to completing our explanation of the decline of bloodletting, clarity about the nature of this innovation will help us understand why the collapse of chimbuki medicine not only preceded, but was, in fact, a *precondition* for the rise of the germ theory.

6

Ignaz Semmelweis and the Adoption of Etiological Concepts of Disease

Philosophy is the struggle against the fascination that forms of speech exert over us.
—*Ludwig Wittgenstein (1958)*

On Friday, November 2, A.S. was admitted to the Hospital and delivered of a female infant, which had apparently died two or three weeks previously . . .. A.S. was a married woman, but exhibited evident signs of syphilis, and to this infection the death *in utero* was probably due. On the following day, Saturday, one of the assistant doctors in the Hospital made a postmortem examination of the fetus, removing the uterus and other organs, and being thus occupied probably for some hours.

On Sunday, November 4, K.M. entered the Hospital in the second stage of labor. Age 22; unmarried; primipara [first delivery] . . .. She had had labor pains to a greater or lesser extent, since the preceding Thursday, and, being homeless and friendless, she had been exposed to great hardships, and had, on the morning of her admission, walked into Boston from a distance, and then wandered about the streets for hours before she was brought to the Hospital. It so happened that on her admission she was received and first examined by the assistant just mentioned, though subsequently delivered by another person. The baby . . . was born about 4:00 p.m., and a severe laceration of the perineum took place. (Jex-Blake, 1877, p. 23)

Five days later, after great suffering, the young woman, known to us only as K.M., died of a disease that was commonly called childbed fever. What was childbed fever?

I

Childbed fever, also called puerperal fever, typically struck young women within a day or two after delivery; it was usually fatal. One

93

British physician described childbed fever as follows: "The disease . . . is ushered in, from the second to the fourth day of confinement, by shivering, accompanied by acute pain radiating from the region of the uterus, increased on pressure, and gradually extending all over the abdomen, with suppression of lochia and milk, much accelerated pulse, furred tongue, great heat of skin, and a peculiar pain in the sinciput [forehead]. [Patients usually have] short breathing, their knees drawn up, and great anxiety of countenance" (Miller, 1848). It is difficult, today, to appreciate the magnitude of the suffering inflicted by this disease in earlier ages. In the eighteenth and nineteenth centuries, it claimed tens of thousands of women each year. While the disease was always of serious concern, in some years, it seemed to sweep through Europe in great epidemics.

In early nineteenth-century Europe, nearly half of all live births were to single mothers, most of whom, like K.M., being "homeless and friendless," ended up delivering in charity hospitals. It was generally known that women who delivered in these facilities were much more likely to die of childbed fever than were those who delivered at home. One physician estimated that about 1 in 29 women who delivered in the hospitals died of childbed fever, whereas, among those who delivered at home, the mortality rate seemed to be only about 1 in 212 (Landau, 1875, p. 151). There was considerable variation in mortality from one hospital to another. Over intervals of a few weeks, some smaller institutions reported mortality approaching 100 percent. The Maternité in Paris may have had the highest sustained mortality of any large institution: between 1861 and 1864, almost one-fifth of all deliveries ended fatally for the mother (DeLacy, 1989, p. 538).

Childbed fever, like every other disease, was ascribed to a range of possible causes. Accounts of childbed fever usually included many, often thirty or more, possible causes, and of course, these causes invariably included the violation of various moral and social norms. In the late eighteenth century, Charles White, a prominent British obstetrician, observed that childbed fever could arise when the "tightness of stays and petticoat bindings, and the weight of the pockets and of the petticoats" press the intestines and block excretion "thereby forcing the body to reabsorb its own wastes." Other causes were said to include a sedentary inactive life, improper diet, the attendance of numerous friends in a small room, a large fire, air "rendered foul and unfit for respiration," strong liquors mixed with warm water, too many coverings, stagnation of lochia in the womb, damp and close houses, want of cleanliness, the ascension of miasmas from families living below, or hospital miasmas. Moreover, White feared that the disease could also be caused through "violence by instruments or by the hands in delivery" (White, 1773, pp. 2–11).

A German contemporary of White's ascribed the disease to rough treatment, the retention of suppression of menstruation, chilling, cold drinks, depressing passions, the inhabitation of damp or wet dwellings, and the suppression of breast or abdominal-genital secretions. He observed that once the disease began, it could spread by contagion. He warned that it could also be conveyed by secretions—especially genital secretions—from ill individuals, and that a contagium could be generated when many patients were crowded together without adequate ventilation. He cautioned against sharing bathtubs, lavatories, and underwear (Schönlein, 1832, pp. 266f, 284–89, 325).

Somewhat later, in 1845, a British physician observed that, in different cases, childbed fever had been traced "to difficult labor; to inflammations of the uterus; to accumulation of noxious humors, set in motion by labor; to violent mental emotion, stimulants, and obstructed perspiration; to miasmata, admission of cold air to the body, and into the uterus; to hurried circulation; to suppression of lacteal secretion; diarrhea; liability to putrid contagion from changes in the humors during pregnancy; hasty separation of the placenta; binding the abdomen too tight; sedentary employment; stimulating or spare diet; [or to] fashionable dissipation" (Waddy, 1845). Physicians frequently noted the obvious fact that childbed fever was especially prevalent in the charity maternity hospitals where most of the patients were unwed women—this provided a ready explanation for the relatively higher incidence of disease in these facilities.

As with any fever or inflammation, the usual treatment for childbed fever was the antiphlogistic regimen. One British physician described the treatment he preferred:

> I immediately order eight or a dozen leeches to be scattered over the abdomen, and to be followed by a linseed or bran poultice; the vagina to be washed out with tepid water, and, if the lochia be fetid, an injection of chloride of soda used; large doses of Calomel [a mercury compound] and opium to be given every three hours, and beef-tea administered at intervals; the calomel to be pushed to approaching ptyalism [poisoning]: when this commences, the calomel to be remitted. Should the pain not yield quickly under these means, I either apply more leeches, or, if the strength will not allow of them,

make use of the turpentine poultice; the effect of this last is in many cases almost magical. (Miller, 1848)

A few years later, an American obstetrician recommended this treatment:

> The prompt abstraction of blood is called for; take from the arm from twelve to thirty ounces [about one to three pints], depending, of course, on the urgency of the case, and in order that there may be nothing equivocal in the impression made upon the system, bleed from a large orifice, let there be a bold and full stream; in one word, make your patient faint; [fainting] will more readily be accomplished by placing the patient in the sitting position . . . The next indication will be a free action of the bowels . . .. We have an important adjuvant in blisters, after the intensity of the disease is somewhat broken; instead, however, of placing them on the abdomen, I greatly prefer applying them on the internal surface of the thighs, immediately over the femoral arteries. (Bedford, 1868, p. 183)

An editor of *Lancet* gave this account of treatment for childbed fever in the Vienna charity maternity facility: "They employed in most cases, immediately on the commence of the disease, repeated venesection, the application of leeches, emollient cataplasms [medicated towels spread over the skin], emollient clysters [enemas]; at a later period blisters, with the corresponding internal remedies; in some cases calomel and other celebrated remedies; and in some, where gastric affections at first predominated, emetics" (Editor, 1824, p. 88). In Vienna, in addition to massive local and general bloodletting, treatment usually involved blistering. One physician recorded that corpses from the Viennese maternity facility usually arrived in the morgue with enormous open sores on the interiors of the thighs from the blistering agents that had been applied in the attempt to remove heat and poisons from the body (Gester, 1847, p. 477).

II

The charity maternity facility in Vienna was the largest such facility in Europe. Approximately five thousand women gave birth there each year. Since it was impossible for a single professor to supervise such an enormous facility, it was divided into two sections. Each section was supervised by a professor of obstetrics, and day-to-day operations were managed by an assistant—a sort of head resident. The assistant was expected to examine the patients each morning in preparation for the professor's rounds, to assist in obstetrical procedures, to supervise difficult deliveries, and to teach the obstetrical students both by conducting demonstrative autopsies in the morgue and by leading afternoon rounds in the clinic. He was also responsible for the clerical records of his section. The first section provided obstetrical training for medical students; midwives were trained in the second section. In 1846, the professor in charge of the first section of the Vienna facility, the section for medical students, was Johannes Klein. On July 1 of that year, a Hungarian named Ignaz Semmelweis became Kline's assistant in the first section. Semmelweis was twenty-eight years of age. He had recently completed his MD degree, and he intended to specialize in obstetrics.

Upon assuming his responsibilities in the first section, Semmelweis was immediately confronted by the horrible reality of childbed fever. He quickly became aware that the mortality rate in his section averaged about three times that of the midwives' section (Semmelweis, 1861, p. 64). Semmelweis reported that this difference led hospital personnel to behave disrespectfully toward the physicians associated with the first section and that for him life soon became unbearable (Semmelweis, 1861, p. 86). He assumed that the difference in mortality must be due to some difference between the two sections, and he immediately began taking steps to make the sections alike in every possible way. He considered such factors as diet, delivery techniques, and even the access route of the priest who came to perform the final sacraments for dying patients. Not believing that any of these measures could account for the higher morality in his section, he described himself as like a drowning person grasping for straws (Semmelweis, 1861, p. 87). Not surprisingly, in spite of his best efforts, the horrible death rate continued.

Then, in the course of performing an autopsy, a Viennese professor of forensic pathology named Jakob Kolletchka sustained a minor wound from a scalpel that was being used in the autopsy. Kolletchka became sick and soon died. As usual, the cadaver was examined. Since Kolletchka had been Semmelweis's friend, Semmelweis read the protocol of the autopsy. He immediately recognized that the pathological remains in Kolletchka's cadaver resembled those in the cadavers of the maternity patients who died of childbed fever. This recognition proved to be a turning point in Semmelweis's understanding of the disease. He later gave the following account of his thinking:

Kolletschka contracted lymphangitis and phlebitis in the upper
extremity . . .. He died of bilateral pleurisy, pericarditis, peritonitis,
and meningitis . . .. But the maternity patients [who died of childbed fever] also had lymphangitis, peritonitis, pericarditis, pleurisy,
and meningitis . . .. Day and night I was haunted by the image
of Kolletschka's disease and was forced to recognize, ever more
clearly, that the disease from which Kolletschka died was identical to that which had claimed so many maternity patients . . .. The
cause of Kolletschka's death was known; it was the wound by the
autopsy knife that had been contaminated by cadaverous particles.
Not the wound itself, but contamination of the wound by the cadaverous particles caused his death . . .. I was forced to admit that
if his disease was identical with the disease that killed so many
maternity patients, it must have originated from the same cause
that brought it on in Kolletschka. In Kolletschka, the specific causal
factor was the cadaverous particles that had been introduced into
his vascular system. I was compelled to ask whether cadaverous
particles had been introduced into the vascular systems of those
patients whom I had seen die of this identical disease. I was forced
to answer affirmatively.

Because of the anatomical orientation of the Viennese medical
school, professors, assistants, and students have frequent opportuni-
ties to touch cadavers. Ordinary washing with soap is not sufficient
to remove all adhering cadaverous particles. This is proven by the
cadaverous smell that the hands retain for a longer or shorter time.
In the examination of pregnant or delivering maternity patients,
the hands, contaminated with cadaverous particles, are brought
into contact with the genitals of these women, creating the possibility of resorption. With resorption, the cadaverous particles are
introduced into the vascular systems of the patients. In this way,
maternity patients contract the same disease that killed Kolletschka.
(Semmelweis, 1861, p. 87f)

Semmelweis knew that student midwives, who were trained in the
second section of the maternity facility, did not conduct autopsies,
and he saw immediately that this could explain why patients in the
second section were healthier. In May 1847, Semmelweis began requiring all the personnel in his section to wash thoroughly in a solution of chlorinated lime. The washings were intended to remove the
cadaverous material from their hands. By the end of the month, the
mortality rate in his section fell to about one percent, the same level
maintained in the midwives' section—he was convinced that he was
on the right track.

Over the next several months, new outbreaks of childbed fever
convinced Semmelweis that the disease could arise not only from

cadaverous material, but from *any* decaying animal-organic substance. For example, he found that the disease could be caused by discharges from open wounds or by organic matter retained on hospital linens, on instruments, or on the hands of surgeons. Moreover, he concluded that, in addition to being conveyed to a maternity patient, decaying organic matter could be generated in the birth canal itself as a result of tissue damage in delivery or when fluids or tissue fragments were retained after delivery. He inferred that such events accounted for the one percent mortality experienced in the midwives' section—such accidents could prove fatal even without decaying organic matter being conveyed to the patient from external sources. Expanding his original hypothesis in these ways led Semmelweis to the conclusion that *every* case of childbed fever was due to contamination by decaying animal-organic matter.

In May 1850, Semmelweis presented a lecture in which he advanced this new concept of the disease—every case of childbed fever was caused by decaying organic matter. So long as Semmelweis had only advocated disinfectant measures, the reaction to his work was simply that he had said nothing new. British and American obstetricians, who believed that childbed fever could be contagious, had long recommended similar measures as a means of preventing the disease from being conveyed by medical personnel (Semmelweis, 1861, pp. 8–12). However, the reaction to his 1850 lecture was strikingly different. Now, rather than merely dismissing his recommendations as unoriginal, the respondents immediately rejected as false his claim that every case of the disease shared a common cause. As physicians throughout Europe heard about his lecture, more than a dozen reacted in just this way (Semmelweis, 1861, pp. 32–38). To be sure, some respondents thought they agreed with Semmelweis, but in fact, there was much more agreement between his opponents and his supporters than there was between Semmelweis himself and those who claimed to agree with him. The crucial difference was how seriously respondents took his claim that *every* case of childbed fever shared a common cause. Respondents either failed to see that he had made this claim—in which case they may have thought they agreed with him—or they saw that he made this claim and they rejected it. No one seems to have been persuaded by his lecture; no one seems to have agreed with what he maintained. One Viennese obstetrician, Eduard Lumpe, felt that, while Semmelweis's claim had not been adequately demonstrated, it could not be completely discounted either; he observed that the medical profession must "wait and [meanwhile] wash" (Lumpe, 1850, p. 398).

Unfortunately, Semmelweis soon encountered resistance of another kind. As it happened, his work came at a time ill suited to the dispassionate appraisal of new ideas. In 1850, when he delivered his lecture, the Austro-Hungarian Empire was still reeling from the revolutions of 1848, and Hungary, Semmelweis's homeland, was in open revolt against the ruling Viennese Hapsburgs. The conservative senior members of the medical faculty mistrusted all foreigners—including, no doubt, the Hungarian Semmelweis. For reasons that were probably more political than scientific, Semmelweis was obliged to leave his post in the Viennese maternity facility. He returned to his native city of Budapest where he managed to find employment in a small maternity facility. Once again, as in Vienna, he dramatically reduced the incidence of childbed fever in his facility. Yet, in spite of his continuing successes and even though some physicians accepted the practice of chlorine washings, his new concept of the disease found no supporters.

Through these years, Semmelweis himself published nothing; he relied on accounts and letters by students and by other professors to disseminate his ideas. As one might expect, his ideas were often misrepresented and misunderstood. Then beginning in 1858, nearly ten years after his initial discovery, he published a book and a few other accounts of his work. But these publications contained nothing new beyond his 1850 lecture, and they were largely ignored. The medical community was simply unable to accept the notion that every case of childbed fever had the same one cause. This idea seemed absurdly wrong, and almost no one was convinced. In frustration, Semmelweis wrote a series of open letters denouncing the obstetricians of Europe as murders. Of course, this tactic only intensified the problem, and Semmelweis was isolated and ignored.

By this time, Semmelweis had married Maria Weidenhoffer, a daughter of Budapest shopkeepers, who was more than twenty years younger than Semmelweis. Semmelweis's progressively more strident attacks on the unyielding medical profession may have embarrassed his shopkeeper in-laws and shocked his medical colleagues. Now in his midforties, Semmelweis may also have begun showing signs of mental instability. According to one frequently repeated anecdote, in July 1865, when Semmelweis was called upon to make a routine report in a meeting of the Pest College of Medical Professors, "He rose, took a piece of paper from his trousers pocket and, to the stupefaction of those present, began to read the text of the midwives' oath" (Gortvay and Zoltán, 1968, p. 187). At least as recounted in this anecdote, Semmelweis's behavior seems to have been seriously inappropriate, and the event is universally taken as evidence that he was losing his mind (Wootton, 2007, p. 217). However, this anecdote first appeared in print seven years after the purported event; its author was not himself present at the meeting, and there is no corroboration for the story. In fact, while Semmelweis's name appears twice in the official minutes of the July meeting, there is no indication that his behavior was in any way unusual. Three days after the meeting, following official protocol, Semmelweis formally applied for an increase in salary. The increase was approved both by the medical faculty and by the university administration (Carter et al., 1995, pp. 258–59). Moreover, at about the same time, Semmelweis was reappointed to the minor post of secretary–treasurer for the Pest medical society. These developments are hard to understand if his behavior had, in fact, been as seriously inappropriate as the anecdote suggests. The story may be based on some true occurrence, but it probably gives a false impression of what actually happened. Looking back from our point of view, more than a century and a half after the events in question, it is impossible to be sure whether Semmelweis was becoming insane and, if so, of the exact nature of his disorder.

In any case, at the end of July 1865, Semmelweis, his wife, and an unweaned infant daughter left Budapest, supposedly to vacation at a spa in Germany. They were accompanied by one of Semmelweis's assistants and by one of Maria's uncles. After an overnight train ride, the party was met in Vienna by Ferdinand Hebra, a professor and former friend from the Vienna medical school. After depositing Maria and the baby at Hebra's home, Semmelweis was persuaded to make a brief tour of what was purported to be Hebra's private sanitarium (Carter et al., 1995, p. 261). However, following a plan that had been arranged in advance, Hebra and Maria's uncle took Semmelweis directly to a Viennese public insane asylum, where he was to be committed. Unknown to Semmelweis, Maria's uncle had carried a commitment order from Budapest; it had been signed by three Hungarian physicians at least one of whom was known to be Semmelweis's personal enemy—none were psychiatrists. Once Semmelweis realized what was happening, he struggled to escape. He was beaten into submission by the asylum guards, forced into a straitjacket, and locked in a basement cell. A later autopsy disclosed that the beating had resulted in massive internal injuries (Carter et al., 1995, p. 268). His untreated wounds became infected, and on August 13, 1865, less than two weeks after he was committed, Semmelweis died.

Semmelweis was buried in Vienna on August 15, 1865. (His remains were later moved to Budapest.) Only a few persons attended the funeral services; most of those in attendance were from the Vienna General Hospital and among them were two brothers, Karl and Gustav Braun, who were Viennese obstetricians and among Semmelweis's bitterest opponents. From Budapest, only Semmelweis's friend Lajos Markusovsky attended the funeral. Not one family member, not one in-law, not one colleague from the University of Pest was in attendance. Semmelweis's wife later explained her own absence on the grounds that, after her husband was committed, she became so ill that she had been unable to leave her bed for six weeks (Carter et al., 1995, p. 268f).

A few Viennese medical periodicals included brief notices of Semmelweis's death. Two periodicals promised to provide longer eulogies in later issues, but the promised eulogies never appeared. The Budapest periodical *Orvosi Hetilap* (*Medical Weekly*), edited at the time by Lajos Markusovsky, contained a brief notice of Semmelweis's death. Remarkably, since Markusovsky had himself attended the funeral, the notice indicates that Semmelweis had been taken to Vienna on July 20 and had been buried there on August 16—both dates were wrong.

Within two weeks of Semmelweis's death, the Hungarian Association of Physicians and Natural Scientists conducted an annual excursion; the group was led by János Balassa, one of the physicians who had signed the order committing Semmelweis to the insane asylum. The association rules specified that a commemorative address be delivered in honor of each member who had died in the preceding year. For Semmelweis, there was no such address; so far as one can judge from the records of the association, his death was never even mentioned. The statutes of the Pest Association of Physicians also required that a eulogy be delivered in honor of each member in the year of his death; in Semmelweis's case, seven years elapsed before this was done.

Semmelweis had two assistants, and after his death, they both applied for his teaching position. However, at the recommendation of János Balassa, a physician named János Diescher was appointed instead. Diescher had once completed a course that qualified him to conduct deliveries, but he had never been trained in obstetrics. The extent to which he followed Semmelweis's principles is clear from what happened to the mortality rate at the Pest maternity clinic: as soon as Diescher took charge, mortality jumped to six percent—six times the rate Semmelweis had consistently maintained. But there were no inquiries and no protests; the physicians of Budapest said nothing. Almost no one—either in Vienna or in Budapest—seemed willing to acknowledge Semmelweis's life and work. "One said nothing of Semmelweis, it was almost as though one was ashamed of his memory" (Benedek, 1983, p. 320).

III

Semmelweis's story has often been told. What is seldom (indeed, almost never) understood or explained is the true nature and significance of his contribution. Discussions of Semmelweis invariably focus on his adoption of chlorine washings. No doubt, disinfection *was* important; after all, it saved lives. But as both Semmelweis and his contemporaries clearly understood, and as few historians today seem to realize, the chlorine washings were only a *consequence* of his real innovation. As he himself explained, "The important difference between my opinion and the opinion of the English physicians [who also advocated disinfection] is this: in every case, without a single exception, I assume only one cause, namely decaying matter, and am convinced of this. The English physicians, while believing that childbed fever can be caused by decaying matter, recognize in addition all the old epidemic and endemic causes that have been believed to play a role in the origin of the disease" (Semmelweis, 1861, p. 37). As we will see, the idea that childbed fever had only one cause enabled Semmelweis to define the term *childbed fever* in a new and profoundly important way. His use of this new kind of definition is the only aspect of Semmelweis's work that is really important to us, *but it is crucial*. And here is why it matters: in one stroke, definitions of the kind Semmelweis adopted not only made bloodletting totally *obsolete* but, more importantly, as we will see in the next chapter, they completely destroyed the foundations of chimbuki medicine. How could a new kind of definition possibly have such profound effects? What could mere definitions have to do with the fall of bloodletting?

In the early decades of the nineteenth century, *childbed fever*, like the name of every other disease, was defined either in terms of symptoms (in the case of childbed fever: intense postpartum fever) or, under the growing influence of pathological anatomy, in terms of various morbid alterations found in the corpses of victims. Anatomical characterizations of childbed fever often focused on inflammation of the uterus. (The most common characterization was in terms of metritis, inflammation of the uterus). This seemed reasonable since the disease seemed obviously associated with the birth process and since autopsies often disclosed morbid alterations in that organ. However, autopsies frequently revealed inflammation in other organs and tissue systems as well: among other forms of inflammation, the pathologists regularly reported finding peritonitis, phlebitis, lymphangitis, pericarditis, and meningitis. According to the fundamental principles of pathological anatomy, this implied that childbed fever was not a single disease but rather a cluster of symptomatically similar diseases, each of which could be seen as an inflammation of some particular organ or tissue system. In the early decades of the nineteenth century, most physicians who wrote on childbed fever adopted some scheme for classifying different cases depending on where inflammation seemed most pronounced. However, other physicians regarded these distinctions as artificial, and, since there were cases in which autopsy revealed no internal morbidity whatsoever, many fell back on a strictly symptomatic characterization. Of course, given the prevailing medical thinking at the time, both fever and inflammation, one or both of which was always present in childbed fever, usually called for bloodletting; it is not surprising that it was the standard therapy.

How did Semmelweis define *childbed fever*? Rather than in terms of symptoms (e.g., intense postpartum fever) or in terms of the inflammation of some organ (e.g., metritis) or of a tissue system (e.g., peritonitis), Semmelweis characterized the disease as "a resorption fever determined through the resorption of decaying animal-organic matter" (Semmelweis, 1861, p. 114). By the unusual word *resorption*, Semmelweis indicated that, in order for the disease to occur, organic matter, which had been secreted or detached from some living organism and had then begun to decay, had been absorbed back (resorbed) into the bloodstream of a victim—either into the bloodstream of the same person who had been the original source of the decaying matter (self-infection), or, more commonly, into someone else. Obviously, this definition was a direct consequence of his belief that every case of childbed fever was due to decaying organic matter. However, by adopting this definition, the relation between childbed fever and decaying organic matter ceased to be a mere empirical generalization and became true *by definition*, the relation became what is called *analytic.* This kind of definition, one in which a disease is defined in terms of its cause, is called an etiological or a causal definition, and such definitions are used extensively in medicine today.

Before we see how etiological definitions undermined bloodletting, we must be clear about two things: first, because he defined *childbed fever* in terms of what he took to be its cause, Semmelweis's definition was definitely etiological; nevertheless, from our point of view today, his definition is not a particularly good one. Childbed fever, which we know, today, as puerperal sepsis, is now classified as a postpartum infection caused by any of a range of different microorganisms, often in combination, and most commonly including Group A streptococci—simply put, it is usually a strep infection (Carter and Carter, 1994, pp. 97–114). Today, no one would think in terms of decaying organic matter being resorbed into a living body. But this difference is inconsequential; as will soon be apparent, for our purposes, that his definition is dated in this way, does not in any way detract from the significance of the *form* of Semmelweis's definition.

Second, Semmelweis was not alone in adopting an etiological definition, and, depending on how one reads the relevant texts, he was probably not even the first to have done so. In 1835, Simon-François Renucci and Philippe Ricord in France and Agostino Bassi in Italy associated scabies, syphilis, and muscardine (a disease of silkworms) with a parasitic insect, a "special ferment," and a minute fungus, respectively (Carter, 2003, p. 25). Each researcher had reason to believe that the cause he identified was universal just as Semmelweis thought that decaying organic matter was the universal cause of childbed fever. In the same year, 1835, James Paget discovered encapsulated worms in human muscle tissue, worms that, by 1860, were recognized as the universal cause of trichinosis. In 1837, Alfred Donné described a parasitic protozoan, *Trichomonas vaginalis*, which seemed to be invariably associated with a particular inflammation of the vagina, and one year later, Angelo Dubini discovered the hookworm parasite. In 1839, a German pathologist, Johann Lucas Schönlein, discovered that favus was always due to a minute fungus, and in the early 1840s, David Gruby, an Hungarian microscopist working in Paris, described this fungus more precisely and traced several other human skin disorders to other minute fungi. Each of these cases led, or could have led, to a more or less explicit etiological definition of the disease in question. So Semmelweis was not alone and may not have been the first to adopt an etiological definition. At about the same time that

Semmelweis recharacterized *childbed fever* etiologically, other similar characterizations were being given for other diseases.

However, there are several reasons why Semmelweis's characterization is especially worthy of our attention: First, his adoption of an etiological definition is unambiguous and can be documented precisely—he knew he was providing a new definition (although he almost certainly did not fully appreciate why his definition was so significant). Insofar as any of the writers mentioned in the previous paragraph actually gave new definitions, their definitions were implicit and the authors' intentions were never fully clear. Second, childbed fever, the disease for which Semmelweis provided an etiological definition and which we now know as puerperal sepsis, was and still remains a profoundly important human disease—indeed, worldwide, it remains today a leading cause of maternal mortality (Carter and Carter, 1994, p. 113f). Third, partly because his approach was unambiguous and because childbed fever was so prominent, Semmelweis's etiological definition profoundly influenced subsequent medical writers—his approach became a central part of the research tradition that ultimately yielded the germ theory of disease. To be sure, all the writers mentioned in the previous paragraph also contributed to this same research tradition, but in the middle decades of the nineteenth century, none of them (indeed, not all of them together) was discussed nearly as frequently as was Semmelweis. Fourth, as we will see in the next chapter, Semmelweis's theory provides an excellent example of the role of science in medicine and of the relation between medical science and therapeutics. Finally (and most importantly), Semmelweis's definition provoked intense debate. As in the Edinburgh bloodletting controversy, the fundamental assumptions and the most fervently held beliefs in any scientific system become most clear in controversy—to understand early nineteenth-century medicine, one must examine these fracture points. However, my use of the Semmelweis account to illustrate the adoption of etiological definitions should not be taken to suggest that he was the only or even the first person to have defined a disease etiologically. For our purposes, priority matters little; it is the nature of the new definitions that is important, not who was the first to employ them.

So how did the adoption of etiological characterizations affect the justification of bloodletting? In the first two chapters, we saw that bloodletting can be explained and justified on at least two levels: it was a means of controlling fever and inflammation, and it was also a means of reinforcing norms (whose violation supposedly led to plethora and thereby to fever and inflammation). Etiological characterizations were absolutely *fatal* to bloodletting on *both* levels. First, as nineteenth-century physicians willingly acknowledged, bloodletting was aimed at, and indeed was truly effective against, *inflammatory symptoms*, which, as we have seen, to nineteenth-century physicians meant the individual disordered states that collectively constituted a disease. The primary targets of bloodletting were fever and inflammation; by definition, fever is elevated body temperature, and inflammation is local heat, pain, redness, and swelling. Bloodletting helped control all of these symptoms. As long as one thought of disease as nothing other than a collection of such disordered states, there was no denying that bloodletting was effective against disease. As we have seen, physicians commonly acknowledged witnessing its effectiveness in their own practices, Pierre-Charles-Alexandre Louis provided a statistical argument that it worked, and even John Bennett, Alison's great antagonist in the Edinburgh controversy, admitted that bloodletting was effective against inflammatory symptoms. However, once a disease is conceived of as something other than symptoms, bloodletting can easily become irrelevant. Because Bennett thought of pneumonia as a sequence of morbid alterations, a sequence that, once set in motion, could not be affected by bloodletting, he could reject bloodletting as useless. (In this limited and indirect sense, and in this sense only, Bennett was approximately correct in thinking that "an improved acquaintance with the pathology of diseases" contributed to the decline of blood-letting.) In the same way, because we now regard childbed fever as a streptococcus infection, an infection that bloodletting cannot affect, we can reject bloodletting as useless. As symptomatic concepts of disease gave way to etiological characterizations, that is, with the rise of causal concepts of disease, bloodletting, which was effective in treating some symptoms but which is generally useless against what are now seen as the causes of symptoms, became almost universally *irrelevant*.[1] Thus, since bloodletting was conceived of as addressing inflammatory symptoms, the new nonsymptomatic concepts of disease deprived bloodletting of this kind of justification.

Etiological characterizations were also fatal to bloodletting insofar as the practice is conceived of as a means of reinforcing norms. Recall Semmelweis's definition of *childbed fever*: "a resorption fever determined through the resorption of decaying animal-organic matter." This definition, like the etiological characterizations that one finds in medicine today, appeals to causes with three common characteristics: the causes are *natural* in the sense that they make no reference to the willful violation of moral or social norms, they are *universal* in the sense that they are stipulated to operate in every instance of the disease, and they are *necessary* in the sense that without them, the disease cannot occur. As we have seen, bloodletting, the central therapy in chimbuki medicine, made sense as a means of reinforcing norms because, by way of plethora, the violation of moral and social norms seemed to be linked to disease and because it also seemed plausible that bloodletting could reduce plethora. For example, gluttony and "fashionable dissipation" were both thought to engender plethora, and plethora could provoke disease; because bloodletting seemed to attack this link, it could be deemed effective. However, once a disease like childbed fever is defined etiologically in terms of one single natural cause, moral transgressions disappear altogether, plethora vanishes from sight, and bloodletting is left without a target. If one defines diseases etiologically, immorality and plethora are eliminated from the disease picture, and bloodletting, however effective it may be against symptoms or even against the results of moral transgressions, at once becomes *irrelevant*. With the rise of causal concepts of disease, disease, its causes, and therefore its treatments became strictly *amoral* and more generally (what we can call) *anormal*. Even if bloodletting happens to discourage or to compensate for gluttony or for fashionable dissipation, it doesn't really matter because such behaviors are no longer part of the disease picture, and therefore reinforcing the norms that forbid such behaviors ceases to have a bearing on treatment. Even if the charity maternity facilities were full of unwed mothers—even if they had been chock full of gluttonous libidinous whores—that could have no direct bearing on the diseases of their inmates or on the treatment those diseases required. Thus, insofar as bloodletting was conceived of as a means of reinforcing norms, the new amoral and *anormal* concepts of disease were again fatal to bloodletting.

We can now understand how bloodletting could have been given up without there ever having been any statistical evidence that it did not work—with the change in concepts of disease, the practice simply became irrelevant. And this enables us to understand how bloodletting could have been given up by the very physicians who saw before their own eyes and who openly acknowledged that it really did accomplish exactly what it was intended to accomplish. One ceased to be interested in inflammatory symptoms per se or even in immoral behavior in and of itself. So even if bloodletting seemed obviously effective against these factors, *they* were no longer of interest and so *it* was no longer of interest. Finally, we can also appreciate how bloodletting could have been given up without any discussion or debate—the whole subject had simply become moot. There was, to be sure, intense debate about how *childbed fever* was to be defined (although, as usual in such cases, most of the disputants seem not to have realized that the issue in question was semantic). Because bloodletting was tied conceptually to the old definition, the debate over that definition carried with it everything that could be said about bloodletting, although bloodletting itself was never once mentioned in the debate. Once the new definitions were adopted, there was nothing left to say about therapeutic bloodletting or about the antiphlogistic regimen in general; whatever benefits bloodletting may have had, the new concepts of disease simply made the practice *irrelevant.*

A conceptual change—a change in the use of disease names, a change in the use of mere *words*, after all—can easily be dismissed as a purely semantic affair, a matter of philosophy, and not something that would necessarily be regarded as a scientific matter. Of course, changes in disease names were ultimately motivated by statistical studies (such as Semmelweis's) and by experimental results (such as Carl Mayrhofer's), but in discussing these efforts, it was (and it remains today) easy to ignore the role of *semantic* issues and to misunderstand their potentially profound ramifications. The French chemist Antoine Laurent Lavoisier astutely observed, "We cannot improve the language of any science without at the same time improving the science itself; neither can we, on the other hand, improve a science without improving the language or nomenclature which belongs to it" (Lavoisier, 1789). But improvements in language and the ramifications of those improvements are easy to overlook and to misunderstand, and so, for decades, Semmelweis's innovation has been misunderstood and the fate of bloodletting has seemed mysterious.

To some extent, Eduard Lumpe, who was probably Semmelweis's most knowledgeable and insightful critic, understood what was happening when Semmelweis advanced his etiological definition of *childbed fever.* In his response to Semmelweis's 1850 lecture, Lumpe said this:

> When one thinks how, since the first occurrence of puerperal fever epidemics, observers of all times have sought in vain for its causes and the means of preventing it, Semmelweis's theory takes on the appearance of the egg of Columbus. I was myself originally overjoyed as I heard the fortunate results of the chlorine washing; like everyone else, I too have had the misfortune to witness many blossoming young women fall before this devastating plague. However, during my two years as assistant in the first section, I observed incredible variations in the incidence of sickness and death. Because of this . . . any other possibility is more plausible than one common and constant cause. (Semmelweis, 1861, p. 32)

From Lumpe's point of view, Semmelweis had trivialized the problem of childbed fever—he had created an egg of Columbus. By redefining *childbed fever*, Semmelweis had simply defined out of existence every case of the disease except those caused by decaying animal-organic matter—he had defined away every case except those that had this one natural cause and that could, therefore, be controlled by chlorine washings. Alone among Semmelweis's many critics, Lumpe saw that Semmelweis had solved the problem of childbed fever by simply redefining it. From Lumpe's point of view, Semmelweis had, in effect, defined away childbed fever. In fact, what Semmelweis had defined away was bloodletting and with it, as we will see in chapter 7, the whole system of chimbuki medicine.

Lumpe came closest, closer perhaps even than Semmelweis himself, to realizing that Semmelweis's innovation was *semantic*, in a sense *philosophical*. In this sense, by the new definitions of which Semmelweis's was typical, philosophy cleared the way for science to advance. Ludwig Wittgenstein characterized philosophy as "the struggle against the fascination that forms of speech exert over us" (Wittgenstein, 1958). The resistance to Semmelweis was the resistance to being required to give up the traditional way of talking about diseases and their causes and to adopt an entirely new system of language. Semmelweis's contemporaries remained "fascinated" by the old forms of speech—fascinated in the sense in which a deer is fascinated (mesmerized) by the headlights of an approaching vehicle. No one, probably not even Semmelweis himself, realized that by redefining diseases in just this way, by verbally connecting a single disease to a single cause and thereby creating a single unambiguous target for therapy, rational therapeutics at last became possible.

IV

I will conclude this chapter with what can be seen as two appendixes, the first having to do with Semmelweis's influence, the second concerning yet another factor that may have played into the decline of bloodletting.

As I mentioned above, one justification for devoting this chapter to Semmelweis's adoption of an etiological definition is that his use of this approach, in contrast to similar innovations by some of his contemporaries, actually influenced subsequent medical writers— later researchers acknowledged having been influenced by his *concept* of childbed fever. By contrast, one of today's many false myths about Semmelweis—a myth that, in spite of having been refuted by at least three different authors, continues to be repeated—is that, after his death, his work was almost completely ignored. For example, Irvine Loudon wrote, "In the twenty years after his death, Semmelweis's name was mentioned only on rare occasions, and usually in uncomplimentary terms" (Loudon, 2000, p. 108). This is simply false. But because of this persisting myth, I must provide some justification for my claim that Semmelweis's use of etiological definitions was influential.

In fact, elsewhere I have identified nearly fifty physicians and researchers who, directly or indirectly, cited Semmelweis positively during the period from his death until the end of the nineteenth century (Carter, 2003, pp. 54–59). In this context, we can review only a few striking examples that indicate how widely he was known and how favorably his work was viewed. During the late 1860s, a year or two after Semmelweis's death, three important Viennese obstetricians: Carl Mayrhofer, Joseph Späth, and A.G.C. Veit, were all converted to Semmelweis's views. All three had originally opposed Semmelweis, but each seems to have become converted, independently, by his own research (Carter, 2003, p. 55). Mayrhofer was particularly noteworthy: he sought, albeit without complete success, to trace childbed fever to infection by what were called vibrions (microorganisms), and through the following decade, he was frequently mentioned together with Semmelweis.

In 1866, F.L. Winckel published an important and widely used textbook on obstetrics. His detailed historical account included a favorable summary of Semmelweis's position (Winckel, 1866, p. 264). Winckel mentioned that Lange of Munich had been among the first to adopt Semmelweis's views. In a long study of diseases of the female sexual organs, published in 1867 (just two years after Semmelweis's death), A.G.C. Veit noted that "the old idea of miasmatic contagion was first challenged by Semmelweis. He taught that childbed fever was a resorption fever occasioned by infection from decaying organic matter. This view is penetrating ever greater circles and, in a short time, will find no more opponents" (Veit, 1867, p. 678). He also noted that, since childbed fever was the result of a septic poison, it was essential to establish the exact nature of the poison, and he mentioned Mayrhofer's work as a possible solution to this problem. In the same year, 1867, W. Roser observed that Semmelweis's concept of childbed fever had become the accepted position among obstetricians and that even many surgeons had been converted to the doctrine (Roser, 1867, p. 20).

One year later, in 1868, Max Boehr published an essay entitled "On the Infection Theory of Childbed Fever and its Consequences for Public Health Officials." The paper, which was originally presented before the Society of Obstetrics in Berlin, drew heavily on Semmelweis's work and conclusions. Boehr noted that Semmelweis's theory "has the characteristics of all good pathological and physiological theories; it provides a unified, clear, and entirely intelligible meaning for a whole series of anatomical and clinical facts and for the disinterested experiences and discoveries of reliable observers during epidemics. None of the earlier or alternative hypotheses or theories regarding the occurrence of childbed fever has this characteristic to the same degree" (Boehr, 1868, p. 403). Boehr noted that in Semmelweis's book, "the superstitions of our predecessors, who believed in unknown cosmic-telluric-atmospheric influences, were dealt a severe blow, as was the belief in miasmata" (Boehr, 1868, p. 404). The same periodical, in reporting the discussion of Boehr's paper, quoted comments by six physicians. Of these, only one is reported as having said anything opposed to Semmelweis's theory; his comment was that "in addition to contagiousness, there are other causes of childbed fever" (Boehr, 1868, p. 433). According to the published report, "Boehr responded that in addition to artificial infection from external sources, he himself recognized only self-infection through foul matter from the patient herself"—which, of course, was exactly Semmelweis's position. This critical comment and Boehr's response are particularly significant since they concerned, directly, the key difference between Semmelweis and his opponents and, indeed, the key difference that makes Semmelweis significant for our purposes. Otherwise, no comments critical of Semmelweis's view were reported in the journal article.

Semmelweis continued to be cited in German, French, and English sources into the 1880s, although by that time (now fifteen years after Semmelweis's death) more recent developments were beginning to eclipse the older work. In 1888, M. Wertheimer wrote, "The earlier theory of the miasmatic nature of [childbed fever], . . . was first put on the right track by Semmelweis. His theory was soon supported, expanded, and confirmed by a series of authors such as Hegar, Buhl, Winckel, Fischer, Veit, [and] Mayrhofer" (Wertheimer, 1888, p. 5f). In 1882, at the very time when, according to what today passes for conventional wisdom, Semmelweis had been completely forgotten throughout Europe, Wilhelm Fischel wrote, "Although long contested, the opinions of the genial Semmelweis . . . have become part of the common property of a whole generation of medical personnel" (Fischel, 1882, p. 1). The phrase, "the genial Semmelweis"—poignant in view of the treatment he received from his peers and of his ultimate fate—appears again in the same year in an obituary for Carl Mayrhofer (r) (1882).

If, in 1867, Veit could claim that Semmelweis's view "is penetrating ever greater circles and, in a short time, will find no more opponents," and Roser could observe that Semmelweis's concept had become the accepted position among obstetricians and many surgeons, if one year later, in 1868, Boehr could say in a professional medical meeting in Berlin (and apparently encounter almost no opposition) that Semmelweis's theory "has the characteristics of all good pathological and physiological theories" in that it provides "a unified, clear, and entirely intelligible meaning" for a whole series of facts and experiences, if, in 1882, Fischel could write that Semmelweis's opinions had "become part of the common property of a whole generation of medical personnel," and if, in 1888, Wertheimer could say that soon after Semmelweis's death, his theory had been "supported, expanded, and confirmed" by a whole series of authors, of whom he named six, if all of this, then how, dear reader, could anyone possibly hold that, in this period, "Semmelweis's name was mentioned only on rare occasions, and usually in uncomplimentary terms"?

The second appendix to this chapter concerns another possible factor in the decline of bloodletting, although this factor can, at best, help us to understand, not why the use of bloodletting declined, but how that therapy was, to some extent, *replaced*. In chapter 2, we saw that bloodletting may have provided a psychological benefit to those who submitted to it. Since current medical theory called for men to be bled more frequently than women, and the wealthy more frequently than the poor, its use on male aristocrats—on *bloods*, as they were called—may have provided a kind of reassurance and confirmation of their power, role, and significance in society. As we saw, anthropologists and such psychologists as Bruno Bettleheim have claimed that just these benefits accrue to male members of other societies in which therapeutic bloodletting is also practiced. If we suppose that this interpretation is correct, one might suspect that as therapeutic bloodletting was abandoned, some other means would be utilized to achieve this same benefit.

Karl Marx pointed out, long ago, that capitalism converts everything, even flesh and blood, into a commodity—everything is given a cash value. Indeed, in 1966, the United States Federal Trade Commission finally made official what had long been true in fact by decreeing that human blood is a commodity. Of course, medical technology has made it possible literally to buy and sell blood or other tissues or organs. As always in capitalism, the value is set by supply and demand. At the time of this writing, according to a quick search on Google, in China, human blood sells for about $12 a pint, whereas, in the United States, the Red Cross, which controls about half the nation's blood supply, charges about $130–$150 a pint. Westerners in serious need of blood, or especially of organs, often find it cheaper and more expeditious to travel to Asia to buy, say, a kidney, than to wait for one to become available at home. Some reject as unethical this practice, which is called transplant tourism, but it flourishes nevertheless.

Thus, by providing a cash equivalent, capitalism obviates the necessity of achieving expiation by actually giving blood. As priests discovered centuries ago, that being who is the object of religious veneration apparently finds cash no less acceptable as an offering than one's own body fluids, and cash is certainly more useful to the officiator—be it the priest or priest-physician. It is, perhaps, more than a coincidence that, depending on how one measures such things, the economic well-being of the medical profession was finally achieved just at about the same time that bloodletting ceased.

In recent decades, Ivan Illich and Thomas McKeowen have pointed out that there is little correlation, either on an individual or a national level, between medical expenditures and health or longevity. We seem willing—eager—to spend virtually any amount of money in the quest for health (the quest for wholeness of mind and body). Our current expenditures on medical care are estimated to exceed 17 percent of our gross national product, with little measurable benefit in respect to reducing morbidity or to extending longevity. From all of this, one must begin to suspect that we are, after all, still being bled—bled in a sense that may no longer be literal but still remains, somehow, more than merely metaphorical. And, of course, as responsibility for morbidity is taken from the individual and assigned to society at large (through, for example, environmental pollution, widespread advertising of such products as cigarettes and soft drinks, the consumption of fast foods, the ever expanding use of pesticides, the use of toxic building materials, and the depletion of the ozone layer), the costs of treatment must also be assumed by society in the form of medical insurance and national health plans. We are collectively guilty of the excesses that are making each of us sick. So be it. Let the staggering costs of expiation be upon us all and, thanks to the national debt, upon our posterity.

So, whatever happened to the psychological benefits of bloodletting? Still stands the ancient sacrifice. The gift on the alter may look like money, but don't be deceived; today's chimbukis have merely transubstantiated your own flesh and blood. The outward economic token is only the sign of an inward and spiritual grace. We now buy expiation with blood money instead of with blood. Bloodletting and its benefits are still alive—it has merely been transmogrified into Medicare.

Note

1.   To be precise, there are relatively rare medical conditions for which bloodletting is still of some use, and some have speculated that by reducing the iron content in the blood, bloodletting may even have some effect in certain infections—but these issues are strictly peripheral to the argument.

7

The Collapse of Traditional Medicine and the Rise of Medical Science

As ideas are preserved and communicated by means of words, it necessarily follows that we cannot improve the language of any science without at the same time improving the science itself; neither can we, on the other hand, improve a science without improving the language or nomenclature which belongs to it.
—Lavoisier (1789)

We have identified two factors that contributed to the decline and fall of bloodletting: (1) in the early nineteenth century, physicians experienced what they referred to as a change in type, a change that, I have suggested, could be explained in terms of the emergence of a new class of patients. Through these decades, physicians encountered proportionally fewer and fewer patients who belonged to the social classes in terms of which the use of bloodletting was traditionally explained and justified; so fewer and fewer patients seemed to require bloodletting, and its use declined accordingly. (2) Diseases were redefined in terms of causes thereby creating a new agenda for medicine.

The new agenda excluded bloodletting in two ways: (1) in chimbuki medicine, diseases were construed as collections of symptoms (disordered states) and treatment focused on these symptoms. Because bloodletting was clearly effective against inflammatory symptoms, it was a prominent and reasonable therapy. By contrast, with the adoption of the new causal concepts, so far as possible each disease was defined in terms of a single universal cause, and it was apparent that treatment could be effective only by addressing that cause; since bloodletting could not do so, it became irrelevant to treatment. (2) In chimbuki medicine, since violations of moral and social norms were regularly included among the numerous possible causes of each disease, treatment could reasonably include measures to reinforce those norms and to correct for the plethoric state that seemed to follow from their violation. Because bloodletting could plausibly be seen as compensating for certain excesses and as reducing plethora, it was a prominent therapy. By contrast, given the new causal concepts, each disease was defined in terms of a single natural cause, and it was clear that the violation of norms had nothing to do with such causes; this made bloodletting irrelevant. The first of these two factors was social; the second, being a consequence of the new etiological definitions, could be seen as semantic or even philosophical. Neither factor entailed a direct experimental nor a statistical refutation of bloodletting, and neither factor was what one might think of as *scientific*. Except in retrospect, neither factor was of a sort that one would expect to hear presented in a medical conference or discussed in a journal article. Both factors were, in effect, *covert* killers of the traditional therapies.

However, the second factor—the rise of causal concepts of disease—counted against more than mere bloodletting. It undermined chimbuki medicine on the most fundamental level, and by doing so, it prepared the way for scientific medical theories. This requires some explanation. The first three parts of this chapter provide background that is necessary in order to appreciate how etiological definitions contributed to this change. First, we will review a few developments in the evolution of the medical understanding of Down syndrome—mongolism,[1] as it was originally called; this will provide an illustration of a kind of medical progress that can easily be overlooked. Second, we will contrast Semmelweis's account of childbed fever with accounts of rabies (hydrophobia as it was commonly called) that were typical of those that appeared in Semmelweis's time. Third, we will briefly introduce some concepts from the philosophy of medicine. All of this will put us in a position, in the fourth and final part of the chapter, to understand the relation between the collapse of chimbuki medicine and the rise of scientific medicine.

I

John Langdon Haydon Down's most interesting and influential paper, "The Ethnic Classification of Idiots," appeared in 1866. In it he wrote, "I have for some time had my attention directed to the possibility of making a classification of the feeble-minded, by arranging them around various ethnic standards" (Down, 1866, p. 212). Down reported having encountered feebleminded persons, born to Caucasian parents, whose physiognomy suggested Malay, Ethiopian, and Aztec origins; however, the most common ethnic pattern and the only one to which he gave extended attention was one he identified as Mongol. According to Down, approximately 10 percent of the feebleminded inmates at the Earlswood asylum, where he worked, were in this category. He was not the first to describe what we now call Down syndrome, and he may not have been the first to use the term *mongoloid* in reference to victims of the disorder (Carter, 2002, p. 530). However, his writings and lectures focused attention on the condition and popularized the use of the term.

In 1899, after examining numerous patients with the disorder, G.A. Sutherland summarized the anatomical abnormalities associated with mongolism and concluded that such a uniform pattern could only be explained by a common cause: "General causes such as parental alcoholism, nervous disease, or insanity in the family, etc., are not likely to produce such an exact type of disease as exists in mongolism. It seems probable that one and the same cause is at work in all cases" (Sutherland, 1899, p. 632). In 1923, T. Halbertsma of Holland described fifteen cases in which only one dizygotic (fraternal) twin was mongoloid; however, he knew of no cases in which mongolism occurred in only one of what appeared to be monozygotic (identical) twins—such twins seemed always to be either both normal or both mongoloid. He concluded that "theories that accept the possibility of an acquired origin during intrauterine life are untenable . . . mongolism has to be regarded as the result of defects inherent in the germ plasm" (Halbertsma, 1923, pp. 351, 353).

By the early 1930s, the observations noted in the previous paragraph were widely known to physicians: first, in mongolism, one observed a striking uniformity of equally striking anatomical abnormalities— abnormalities that seemed to affect virtually every part of the body, and second, while one infant from a pair of dizygotic twins had about the same likelihood of being mongoloid as any baby selected at random, among monozygotic twins either both were mongoloid or neither was. Two theories emerged to explain these observations: first, that mongolism was a rare inheritable trait (or collection of traits)—this was known as the Hereditary Theory. The chief defect in this theory was that the occurrence of the disorder in families was not compatible with what one would have expected on the basis of Mendelian genetics. The second theory was that mongolism could result from some influence (perhaps endocrine imbalance or simple aging) that harmed ova in some way—this was known as the Defective Ova Theory. The defect in this theory was that it seemed incompatible with the observed uniformity of anatomical abnormalities (Carter, 2002, p. 542).

Between 1932 and 1938, three medical researchers suggested, each independently of the others, that mongolism could be due to a chromosomal abnormality such as nondisjunction: the first was Petrus Johannes Waardenburg, a young Dutch scientist (1932); the second was Adrien Bleyer, an American pediatrician (1934); and the last was Guido Fanconi, a Swiss physician (1938). Although Waardenburg was the first to propose nondisjunction, he advanced this hypothesis in a book on inheritable attributes of the eye, and the title of the book did not suggest a connection with mongolism. No one who wrote on Down syndrome seems to have been aware of Waardenburg's conjecture until it was rediscovered in the 1960s (Carter, 2002, p. 547). Franconi also published in a relatively obscure source and was seldom cited. Of the three, Bleyer's conjecture, which appeared in a commonly accessible journal, was by far the most widely known and frequently discussed. Bleyer proposed that the syndrome could arise when—perhaps because of nondisjunction—cells lacked the proper number of chromosomes. If so, "a very early alteration in the germ cell . . . would repeat itself in every cell derived therefrom throughout the entire body" (Bleyer, 1934, p. 348). This could obviously explain the uniform and widespread anatomical abnormalities observed in Down syndrome, as well as the distribution of the disorder among twins. He also noted that this explanation avoided the defects that seemed to count against the Hereditary and the Defective Ova theories.

Unfortunately, in the 1830s, existing experimental techniques were not sufficiently sophisticated to allow the chromosomal hypothesis to be confirmed; twenty years elapsed before Bleyer's conjecture could be tested. In the meantime, it came to be known as the Mutation Theory. This title suggested, falsely, that Bleyer was thinking of what is now called a point mutation rather than of chromosomal nondisjunction, and any specific point mutation occurs far too seldom to account for the observed frequency of Down syndrome. Largely due to this misrepresentation, Bleyer's conjecture was universally rejected. In 1959, Jerome Lejeune, Marthe Gautier, and Raymond Turpin discovered that Down syndrome was due to the particular nondisjunction now known as trisomy 21. In a sense, the discovery vindicated Bleyer, but by then, both Bleyer and his astute conjecture, which had been consistently misinterpreted and misrepresented, had been all but forgotten (Carter, 2002).

Since its confirmation by Lejune, Gautier, and Turpin, the explanation of Down syndrome as a form of nondisjunction has been expanded and elaborated by a whole series of researchers. In 1959, the same year in which Down syndrome was conclusively shown to be trisomy 21, Turner syndrome and Klinefelter syndrome were also associated with specific chromosomal abnormalities. One year later, trisomies 13 and 18 were described. "By 1970 over 20 different human chromosomal disorders were known. The development of chromosomal banding in 1970 markedly increased the ability to resolve small chromosomal aberrations, and so by 1990 more than 600 different chromosome abnormalities had been described" (Connor and Ferguson-Smith, 1997, p. 5).

Who could doubt that these developments constitute progress in medicine? Yet to this day, in spite of the ever-increasing understanding of chromosomal anomalies, not one case of Down syndrome has been averted or corrected; not one life has been saved. If we insist that medical progress is only about reducing morbidity or mortality, then we must conclude that, so far, there has been no significant medical progress in respect to genetic disorders like Down syndrome. But this would clearly be absurd. Medicine obviously involves more than just reducing morbidity. So what is progress in medicine?

There is nothing inherently wrong with measuring the success of physicians' attempts to reduce morbidity and to extend life or with charting that success through history. However, if we take advances in these areas to be the *only* or even the *primary* measure of medical progress in general, we are forced into an unrealistically narrow concept of *medicine*. Progress in reducing morbidity and in extending life is, at best, a consequence, and sometimes a very remote consequence, of progress in *understanding*, and medicine includes understanding. So one cannot assume that progress in medicine means simply progress in control. Yet one occasionally encounters this confusion—David Wootton observed that "deferring death is the main test of medicine's success" (Wootton, 2007, p. 269). Why would one make such an assertion which so obviously ignores much of what is clearly medical success? One reason may be *semantic*. Unlike words that name other sciences (e.g., *physics*, *chemistry*, or *physiology*), we use the word *medicine* to refer both to a body of theoretical knowledge and to the application of that knowledge in the quest for health. (It is as if we were to use *physics* to include both what we now call physics as well as its engineering applications). Because our language does not clearly mark the distinction between medical theory and medical practice, the distinction is easy to ignore.

A second source for this confusion may be, in a sense, *psychological*. Medicine touches every human life, and it is *imminent* in a way that no other scientific endeavor can be. Most of us seek the professional services of physicians several times each year; by contrast, one goes a lifetime without personally soliciting the professional services of a physicist or a geologist. And precisely because medicine is so much a part of our lives, we may fail to think about just what is involved in medical treatment. To be sure, we understand, on some level, that effective treatment is the application of what was once pure medical science. When we visit a physician, we understand, dimly, that the care we receive is based on research that was (in all probability) conducted by some other persons, in some other venues, and at some earlier times; but all we care about, right now, is being healed. Whatever was done in a laboratory that makes the healing possible (i.e., what can be called the pure part of medicine) blends into and seems to derive its significance from, what is going on now, in my current treatment. So because treatment is so often so important to us, it is easy to collapse medicine into treatment, and progress in medicine into success in treatment, that is, progress in keeping patients alive. But as we see from research on Down syndrome, medicine is much more than this. Modern medicine, as Wootton himself acknowledges, is to be defined as "constant improvements in therapy grounded in constantly developing scientific understanding" (Wootton, 2007, p. 227). Exactly. There may be improvements in therapy, but the crucial fact is the constantly developing scientific understanding.

II

How else might one measure progress in medicine? The contrast between the early nineteenth-century conception of rabies and Semmelweis's account of childbed fever will help answer this question. Before the rise of causal definitions, diseases were almost always defined in terms of prominent symptoms. For example, as we have seen, Gabriel Andral defined *hydrophobia* as a complete horror of fluids reaching to such a degree that swallowing becomes almost impossible (Andral, 1832–3, p. 806). However, if hydrophobia is a horror of swallowing, then, as Andral himself emphasized, fully authentic cases could be caused by blows to the throat or by psychological problems as well as by the bites of rabid dogs. Given a symptomatic definition like Andral's, it was logical, inevitable, and *true* to surmise that hydrophobia, or almost any other disease so defined, could be caused in many different ways, and contemporary physicians were entirely comfortable with this way of thinking. However, explanations are typically based on causes, and if a disease is defined in such a way that it can have any number of different causes, general explanations such as those we associate with science become almost impossible. For example, suppose we accept Andral's definition of *hydrophobia*. Given several cases of the disease, the patients will share the prominent symptom of being unable to swallow, but they could differ in virtually every other respect: the individual cases would likely progress and terminate quite differently, therapies effective in some cases might have no effect in others, the epidemiological and anatomical features of the cases could be totally unlike, and so on. Apart from the pathognomonic symptom, there would be no necessary commonalities among the different cases. And, in the absence of common disease phenomena, there could be no general explanations of anything—each case would remain more or less unique.

In such a situation, medicine could only be a kind of art based on the experience and intuitions of the physician, but nothing like science would be possible. In respect to prophylaxis or therapy, the best one could hope for would be recommendations that would sometimes work. One sees exactly the same limitations in understanding and in controlling any symptomatically defined disease. For another example, recall ophthalmia as discussed in chapter 1: given Buchan's symptomatic characterization, what commonalities, other than the symptoms themselves, could possibly be shared among any set of cases of the disease? At best one could treat the common symptoms; that would be done best by some method that works against every form of inflammation, for example, by bloodletting. By contrast, once a disease is defined in terms of a cause, every instance of the disease must, by definition, share that one cause, and this common cause will usually have common effects in each victim and this will result in common disease phenomena, and this, in turn, often makes it possible to give general explanations that apply to *every* case of the disease (as defined etiologically) and, occasionally, it provides a basis for systematic therapy or prophylaxis.

This contrast is stunningly apparent to anyone who compares Semmelweis's account of childbed fever with those of other writers from the same period. In 1843 (four years before Semmelweis began work in the first section of the Viennese maternity facility), Oliver Wendell Holmes, an American physician, wrote an essay on childbed fever in which he strongly urged physicians to use disinfectant measures to avoid spreading the disease (Holmes, 1843). Because of this recommendation, Holmes is often credited with having preceded Semmelweis in seeking the same results for which Semmelweis is sometimes given credit (Wootton, 2007, pp. 211–23). Holmes's essay was based on many reported observations of the occurrence of childbed fever; however, believing as he did, that childbed fever could have an unlimited range of different causes, it was impossible to generalize from the observations, and he explained virtually *nothing* about the disease. Two years later, Eduard Lumpe, who had preceded Semmelweis as an assistant in the first section of the Viennese facility, also published an essay on childbed fever (Lumpe, 1845). Lumpe knew and mentioned almost all the facts that were later available to Semmelweis. However, assuming as he did, that the disease could have an unlimited range of different causes, Lumpe made no attempt to generalize from or to explain these facts. He made interesting observations. He gave beneficial advice (e.g., he noted and endorsed the British use of disinfection), but like Holmes, he explained *nothing* about the disease.

The difference between Semmelweis and everyone else who wrote on the disease, including both Holmes and Lumpe, is the difference between day and night. In their essays, however interesting and however beneficial, Holmes and Lumpe explained almost nothing. By contrast, in addition to practical advice that could reduce the incidence of (what he now called) childbed fever from 10 percent or more to about 1 percent, Semmelweis provided a complete explanatory theory. For example, Semmelweis explained why patients in the midwives' section were healthier than those in the first section, why the mortality rates in the two sections had changed over the years, why women who delivered at home or on the way to the hospital or who delivered prematurely were healthier than those who went full term in the facility, why the disease sometimes appeared within a facility in particular patterns, why it was rare during pregnancy or more than a few days after delivery, why it sometimes appeared to be contagious, why it exhibited seasonal patterns, why it was most prevalent in teaching hospitals, why some nonteaching hospitals had lower mortality rates than others, why the disease appeared with different frequencies in different countries and in different historical periods, why infants never died from childbed fever unless their mothers also contracted the disease, why the mortality rates of infants changed in certain ways, and much, much more. Lumpe knew virtually all of the same facts, but he explained nothing; because of his new concept of the disease, Semmelweis could explain everything.

Those who write on Semmelweis today (and they are legion) seem almost always oblivious of this striking difference between Semmelweis and *all* of his predecessors. Yet, to at least some of his contemporaries, the difference was perfectly clear. Recall Max Boehr's comments in his 1868 lecture: "Semmelweis's theory," he observed, "has the characteristics of all good pathological and physiological theories; it provides a unified, clear, and entirely intelligible meaning for a whole series of anatomical and clinical facts and for the disinterested experiences and discoveries of reliable observers during epidemics. None of the earlier or alternative hypotheses or theories regarding the occurrence of childbed fever has this characteristic to the same degree" (Boehr, 1868, p. 403). The difference can't be described more plainly than that. Twenty years later, in 1888, Max Wertheimer observed that "the earlier theory of the miasmatic nature of [childbed fever—to which, incidentally, both Holmes and Lumpe subscribed], . . . was first put on the right track by Semmelweis. His theory was soon supported, expanded, and confirmed by a series of authors such as Hegar, Buhl, Winckel, Fischer, Veit, [and] Mayrhofer" (Wertheimer, 1888, p. 5f). Wertheimer understood perfectly *both* that Semmelweis's account of childbed fever marked genuine progress in understanding the disease *and* that Hegar, Buhl, Winckel, Fischer, Veit, and Mayrhofer made yet further progress by building on Semmelweis's work.

Between them, in the two quotations at the end of the previous paragraph, Boehr and Wertheimer identified two important features of medical progress (and neither quotation, by the way, so much as mentioned the chlorine washings or the other prophylactic measures that, in the eyes of today's historians, are the sum total of Semmelweis's contribution): first, progress requires new theories that provide better and more extensive explanations than were provided by earlier theories, and second, progress requires theories that can be tested, elaborated, and expanded by other researchers. In short, medical progress is a kind of collaborative effort at expanding and perfecting explanatory theories of disease. We are now prepared to generalize these conclusions but, in doing so, it will be helpful to have available a few concepts from the philosophy of science to which we now turn.

III

If we think of medicine as a pure science, then medical progress will be like progress in any pure science. How are we to understand scientific progress? In an attempt to characterize scientific progress in general, Imre Lakatos introduced the concept of scientific research programmes (Lakatos, 1968). In simple terms, a research programme comprises a sequence of progressively stronger scientific theories that exploit shared methods to explain a specific subject matter. Thus, a research programme is a kind of cooperative activity focusing on the elaboration of scientific theories as a means of explaining observations. This, of course, very much resembles how, half a century in advance of Lakatos, Boehr and Wertheimer described the medical developments that followed and were built on Semmelweis's work. On the basis of their remarks, one could say that Semmelweis launched a scientific research programme.

Two aspects of research programmes require further explanation: first, the notion of a cumulative effort, that is, the notion that various people can successively elaborate and expand a research programme, and second, the notion of scientific theories. As Wertheimer's comment illustrates, over time, many people may and usually do contribute to a research programme. How does one decide who, exactly, is contributing to which programme? For practical purposes, this can be resolved by examining *citations*. There is no need for citations when drawing on shared background knowledge. References are required only for claims that are not universally acknowledged or that are recognized as part of the proprietary domain of some individual or group. Moreover, a new idea or method contributes to a continuous research programme only if others adopt it, and one expects such borrowing to be acknowledged in citations. Thus, a research programme can be regarded approximately as a collection of works linked through citations, and one can individuate programmes by constructing citation indexes (Carter, 2003, p. 4). For example, directly or indirectly, Ignaz Semmelweis, Robert Koch, Louis Pasteur, and even Sigmund Freud and John Langdon Down were all connected to one another through a web of citations. In a sense, therefore, all of these individuals can be seen as working within the common research programme that we call modern medicine. By

126

contrast, William Buchan, Oliver Wendell Holmes, or (to take a more fanciful example) the great sixteenth-century speculator, Girolamo Fracastoro, for all the good that they may have achieved, are not so linked and, therefore, using our criterion, they are not part of this research programme.

While we can separate and identify research programmes by citation indexes, the programme itself is the sequence of theories that emerge from the use of shared methods. In a sense, theories constitute pure science, and science progresses by generating ever more successful theories. So what is a theory in this sense? And what does it mean to say that a theory is successful? In ordinary discourse, we use the word *theory* loosely to refer to any conjecture about how things work. In science, the term is used in a narrower sense, the sense exemplified by such phrases as "the theory of evolution," "the kinetic theory of gasses," "the theory of relativity," or, "the germ theory of disease." In this sense, theories can be regarded as sets of laws, where the term *law* refers approximately to a syntactically and semantically general statement with empirical content that is embedded in a theory (Van der Steen and Kamminga, 1991, p. 445f). This requires some illustration and explanation. In the physical sciences, theories are often stated quite precisely, and some can be cast in purely mathematical notation. When this happens, the theory may resemble an axiom system such as Euclidian geometry. As an example, the kinetic theory of gases can be thought of as the set of all the consequences of the following four propositions: "(1) a pure gas consists of a large number of identical molecules separated by distances that are great compared to their size. (2) The gas molecules are constantly moving in random directions with a distribution of speeds. (3) The molecules exert no forces on one another between collisions, so between collisions they move in straight lines with constant velocities. (4) The collisions of molecules with the walls of the container are elastic; no energy is lost during a collision" (Oxtoby and Nachtrieb, 1990, p. 104). In the preceding quotation, the first statement can be viewed as a definition, but statements two, three, and four have the properties identified in our definition of *law*: they are syntactically and semantically universal, they have empirical content, and they are embedded in a theory. From these general statements, one can derive, mathematically, the familiar truths of the kinetic theory (e.g., Charles' Law, Boyle's Law, etc.). Given our definition of *theory*, it is apparent that laws and theories are mutually dependent—neither is possible in the absence of the other.

Now, what is the purpose of a scientific theory? As one could infer from what has already been said, it is to provide explanations. Norwood Russell Hansen observed that the purpose of a theory is to provide "an intelligible, systematic, conceptual pattern for the observed data. The value of such a pattern lies in its capacity to unite phenomena which, without the theory, are either surprising, anomalous, or left totally unnoticed" (Hansen, 1963, p. 44). This, of course, is perfectly exemplified by Max Boehr's statement that Semmelweis's theory "has the characteristics of all good pathological and physiological theories; it provides a unified, clear, and entirely intelligible meaning for a whole series of anatomical and clinical facts and for the disinterested experiences and discoveries of reliable observers during epidemics" (Boehr, 1868, p. 403). Boehr's comment also suggests one standard by which the quality or the success of theories can be appraised: other things equal, the more a theory explains the better it is.

Obviously, much more could be said about the extremely rich concepts of scientific laws, theories, and research programmes; in this context, however, these brief remarks must suffice. We must now apply these general observations to the collapse of traditional medicine and to its replacement by medicine as we now know it.

IV

Beginning at least as early as the sixteenth century, and possibly long before, numerous persons had speculated about the causes of infectious diseases, and some of this speculation involved what were sometimes called viruses or seeds—undetectable entities by which, it was supposed, diseases could be conveyed (Wootton, 2007, p. 124f). Among these speculators was Girolamo Fracastoro, whose name is, even today, occasionally mentioned by historians as a precursor of the germ theory of disease. But before the nineteenth century, there were no theories of disease in the sense in which *theory* is defined in the preceding section, and the speculators did not contribute to a research programme because they were not cited and their speculations were not expanded or elaborated by anyone. Each speculator, for example, Fracastoro, had his own opinions, but his speculations, however interesting they may now be to antiquarians, do not qualify as a theory and they were never taken up into the research programme that we now know as medicine. In contrast, Semmelweis's account can be stated in such a way as to meet, precisely, our definition of *theory*, and it was not only cited but "supported, expanded, and confirmed by a series of authors such as Hegar, Buhl, Winckel, Fischer, Veit, [and] Mayrhofer" and their work, in turn, was not only cited but supported, expanded, and confirmed by another series of authors, and this series included the most famous bacteriologists of the nineteenth century: Edwin Klebs, Robert Koch, and Louis Pasteur (Carter, 1985a). In short, Semmelweis's account was an explanatory theory (and, indeed, a good one), and even though his account did not involve germs (indeed, he rejected the notion that microorganisms could be causally involved in childbed fever [Semmelweis, 1861, p. 249]), it became part of a shared research programme that ultimately included the germ theory of disease (Carter, 2003). And what, exactly, is the germ theory of disease? If it is truly a scientific theory, it must be possible to state it in such a way that it meets the definition that we have discussed.

In discussing the germ theory, David Wootton identifies Felix Platter (1563–1614) as possibly the earliest "proper germ theorist" on the grounds that, in the case of plague and syphilis, he rejected spontaneous generation, held that each disease was due to a living germ, and insisted that the germ was a necessary condition—a *sine qua non*—for onset of the disease (Wootton, 2007, pp. 124–29). Be this as it may, the role of microorganisms in disease was not actively investigated until the second half of the nineteenth century. By the 1870s, anthrax, relapsing fever, and some wound infections had been associated with specific microorganisms, but the exact nature of the association remained unclear and most physicians had not yet accepted the notion that diseases could be caused by germs (Carter, 2003, pp. 92–95). In 1875, in discussing a group of microorganisms that included bacteria, Edwin Klebs identified what he called *Grundversuche* (Klebs, 1875–6, p. 376f), a term that, in light of how he uses it, could be translated as "fundamental assumptions." While Klebs's account is far from clear, the *Grundversuche* can be read as including the following claims: (1) all diseases are caused only by bacteria, (2) distinguishable diseases are always caused by distinguishable bacteria, (3) bacteria never arise spontaneously, and (4) healthy animals are free from all pathogenic bacteria. Klebs described the *Grundversuche* as simplifying assumptions, assumptions that were to be invoked prior to any attempt to demonstrate disease causation. He claimed that this approach was based on the usual way of giving explanations in the physical sciences, and, while he did not use these terms, the *Grundversuche* can be regarded as laws that, when taken together, meet our definition of a scientific theory; as such they constitute what may be the earliest explicit scientific theory of disease. Klebs realized that, as with laws in the physical sciences, one or another of the *Grundversuche* may be literally false or at least impossible to verify, but he also saw that this was no obstacle to using them as a basis for explaining disease.

We come now to the crucial question of this chapter: what would *late* nineteenth-century medicine (or perhaps even medicine today) have been like if chimbuki medicine had not collapsed *before* germs were recognized as causes of disease? Suppose, in the 1890s, physicians had still thought of diseases symptomatically. For example, suppose such physicians had continued to think of hydrophobia as such a complete horror of fluids that swallowing was impossible. Then, thanks to the work of people like Louis Pasteur and Robert Koch, in addition to blows to the throat, psychological disorders, and the bites of rabid dogs, nineteenth-century physicians might have come to recognize streptococcus infections, that is, invading bacteria, as yet another possible cause of hydrophobia (e.g., one could have such an intensely sore throat that the idea of swallowing is absolutely abhorrent). This situation may be made a bit more plausible if we think of Oliver Wendell Holmes or of Eduard Lumpe (or indeed of virtually any of the many respondents to Semmelweis's 1850 lecture) both of whom recognized some sort of contagion, often spread by physicians, as one possible cause among the many others that could bring on childbed fever. What would have happened if medicine, while still clinging to symptomatic concepts of disease, had accepted germs as possible causes of disease? There is, after all, nothing in the notion of germs that forces one to abandon symptomatic definitions in favor of causal ones. (Indeed, this is approximately our situation, today, in respect to what is called the common cold). So what would have happened if, at the time germs were being accepted as causes, the symptomatic concepts of chimbuki medicine were not already being given up in favor of causal concepts of disease? Perhaps *nothing of any importance would have happened!* And by this I mean that physicians may very well have been left with exactly the same hopeless confusion that they already faced in the 1820s—a confusion in which, apart from symptoms, there were no necessary commonalities among cases of any given disease, and in which, therefore, there could still have been no general explanations and no scientific theories. It is entirely imaginable that, even after recognizing germs as possible causes of diseases, physicians could have continued to think in terms of symptomatic concepts and of multiple causes. In short, *germs could have been seen as yet one more possible kind of cause.* This would have left chimbuki medicine essentially unchanged—an art, perhaps, but definitely not a science.

Why, under these conditions, could medicine not have become a science? For the simple reason that prior to adopting causal definitions of diseases (i.e., prior to the collapse of chimbuki medicine), nothing like the germ theory of disease would have been even conceivable. Suppose we take Klebs's *Grundversuche* as a reasonable approximation of the germ theory of disease. Among their numerous consequences, the *Grundversuche* entail one particularly important notion: if all diseases are caused only by bacteria (*Grundversuch* 1) and if different diseases are caused by distinguishable bacteria (*Grundversuch* 2), it follows that one and only one variety of bacterium will be the only cause of each disease. Once the causal organism is identified, a given disease can then be redefined in terms of this one causal agent. As we have seen, this way of thinking opens the path to scientific explanations and to rational therapy. But this whole way of thinking, this whole way of *talking*, would have been literally inconceivable if diseases were still defined in such a way as to allow (indeed require) a multitude of unrelated causes for each disease. In chimbuki medicine (with its symptomatically defined diseases and their multiple causes), germs could easily have been recognized as yet another kind of cause, but within chimbuki medicine, the mere articulation of the germ theory of disease would have been absolutely, logically impossible. Another way to put this is to say that it was logically necessary for chimbuki medicine to have collapsed before the germ theory of disease, together with all the explanations it provides, could have been even conceivable. In the absence of etiological concepts of disease, even recognizing germs as causes would not have allowed for scientific explanatory theories in which each case of any given disease shares common features with every other case of that disease and in which those commonalities can be explained in terms of the one common cause.

By contrast, once etiological definitions are in place, then theories like the *Grundversuche* can focus attention on a particular range of entities (in the case of the germ theory: bacteria; for genetic disorders: chromosomal and other genetic abnormalities; for deficiency diseases: lack of vitamins, and so forth) within which alone causes are to be sought—causes in terms of which disease commonalities can then be explained. One consequence of this approach is what has been called a monocausal or a monogenic model of disease (Broadbent, 2009). Once adopted, this way of thinking quickly spread through medicine and the quest for specific monocauses has dominated much of medical thinking down to the present time (Carter, 2003). As Kräupl F. Taylor observed in 1979, "The final hope and aim of medical science is the establishment of monogenic disease entities" (Taylor, 1979, p. 21). Why does this quest dominate so much of medical research? Precisely because the identification of such causes—monocauses—is absolutely essential for the explanatory theories that are the hallmark of any science and of scientific medicine in particular.

In articulating the germ theory, directly or indirectly, Klebs cited or was cited by all the famous nineteenth-century researchers including (of course) Ignaz Semmelweis, Joseph Lister, Robert Koch, Louis Pasteur, and lots of other people whose work actually contributed to successive articulations of the germ theory of disease (but, not, so far as I can determine, chimbuki physicians like Buchan, Holmes, Platter, or Fracastoro, the great speculator). Here, we finally have a true research programme focusing on human diseases. Here, we finally have true progress in medicine. The product of this particular research programme, the standard against which success is measured, is the understanding of human diseases. Some of this increased understanding has actually enabled physicians to reduce morbidity and mortality, but much (probably most) of it has not. This is reasonable because, ultimately, like any scientific theory, the germ theory of disease (and the other theories that constitute modern medicine) is about understanding, and not necessarily about engineering. Indeed, as numerous writers have pointed out, much of the credit for this kind of success— the success of lengthening lives—that is usually awarded to the promulgators of the germ theory is *not* actually deserved (McKeown, 1976).

V

We can now draw together some of our conclusions and, in the process see why the collapse of chimbuki medicine was not just antecedent to, but a genuine precondition for, the rise of scientific medicine. One characteristic of modern medicine—scientific medicine—is the use of scientific theories to explain disease. Success in science (and therefore in scientific medicine) stems from the work of various researchers who "support, expand, and confirm" antecedent theories and who thereby contribute to a research programme. The particular theories that medicine uses are theories in which, as far as possible, each disease is associated with a specific cause. We saw this in Klebs's *Grundversuche* where it is assumed that each disease is caused by one and only one species of bacterium. The value of such a theory is clear in Semmelweis's account of childbed fever—it enables one to explain a whole range of observations and, occasionally, to identify effective means of control. So, as far as possible, medicine progresses through the identification, expansion, and elaboration of theories in which each disease is conceived of as having a single cause—a monocause. But how is this to be achieved? It clearly depends on defining diseases in such a way that each will have a single cause, and this is by no means a trivial accomplishment. For example, if diseases are defined symptomatically, most diseases will necessarily have an array of independent causes because most sets of symptoms can come about in more than one way. As we have seen, given symptomatic definitions, cases of a given disease will not necessarily share common qualities, general explanations will be impossible, and there will be no medical science. We see, therefore, that before scientific medicine could be possible, the way had to be opened for diseases to be defined causally so that each disease would have its own unique cause. Another way to put this is to say that chimbuki medicine, a system in which diseases were defined symptomatically and in which, therefore, diseases would not, in general, have unique causes, had to collapse before the causal theories that characterize modern medicine would have been possible. In this way, adopting etiological characterizations undercut, not just bloodletting, but the whole system of chimbuki medicine, and the collapse of chimbuki medicine was not just antecedent to, but was a genuine *precondition* for, the rise of modern medicine.

It is easy to underestimate the *philosophical* difficulty of identifying causes. David Wootton observes that "it is obvious how to set about testing the efficacy of a medical therapy. All that is needed is to take a group of patients with similar symptoms and treat some of them and not others" (Wootton, 2007, p. 144). But clearly, it isn't all that simple. As we saw in chapter 1, by precisely those steps, Philip Crampton confirmed that, in treating ophthalmia, leeches should be applied directly to the conjunctiva. For any such test to be meaningful, one must start out very clear about what one is testing and that will depend crucially on how one defines the disease in question. Indeed, Wootton himself goes on to observe that "in order to test a therapy you need to have a concept of a disease being not a disorderly condition of a particular patient, but a typical condition of many patients, for only then can you be confident that you are comparing like with like" (Wootton, 2007, p. 145). But, given his hospital full of patients with inflamed eyes, Crampton surely *thought* he was comparing like with like. The whole issue is *like in what respect?* And that is precisely why everything depends on getting diseases defined properly. "Before you can count and compare you need to have a conception of disease that makes counting and comparing possible" (Wootton, 2007, p. 283). Precisely.

Wootton observes that in the rise of modern medicine, scientific medicine, "there were conceptual obstacles to be overcome, but it is difficult to see that those obstacles were major ones" (Wootton, 2007, p. 284). But the conceptual obstacles were, indeed, major. We don't find causes as we find shells on a beach. And while microscopes may be useful, they don't even address, much less remove, the philosophical obstacles. Microscopes may reveal anthrax bacilli in the blood of anthracoid sheep, but the presence of the organisms does not establish a causal connection. Causation is ultimately a theoretical relation, so causal claims can never be justified in the absence of a theory (Carter, 2003, pp. 76–89). To say that a set of conditions causes some event is to say that our theories connect the conditions with the event in certain ways—it does not mean that the event is, somehow, once and for all, bonded to those conditions by "cosmic glue" (Hansen, 1963, p. 64)—a sort of glue which the use of a sufficiently powerful microscope will immediately reveal for all to see.

Causation depends as much on our language as on what we can observe. To prove causation, theories are necessary, and for the sort of theories that one uses in medicine, diseases must be suitably defined. In this sense, modern medicine depends as much on advances in philosophy as on anything discovered in a pathology laboratory. In this sense, science advances only when philosophy authorizes and directs it to do so (Mann, 1936).

Note

1. For reasons that now seem obvious, such terms as *mongol, mongolian,* and *mongoloid* are no longer in vogue in reference to the syndrome. However, they were standard in the research I am about to summarize; and since they appear in every quotation, it would be impractical to attempt to avoid them in my discussion.

8

The Current Crisis in Epidemiology

When philosophy paints its grey in grey, then has a form of life grown old. The owl of Minerva spreads its wings only with the coming of the dusk.
—G.W.F. Hegel (1821)

Much of the success that has been achieved in modern medicine has come from the elaboration of a particular way of thinking about disease. This way of thinking, which Robert Koch referred to as the etiological standpoint (Koch, 1901, p. 93), is expressed in a series of theories of disease that constitute a classic research programme exactly as envisioned by Imre Lakatos. In this final chapter, we will consider whether this progress is likely to continue.

I believe Hegel's famous observation is correct: "when philosophy paints its grey in grey, then has a form of life grown old. The owl of Minerva spreads its wings only with the coming of the dusk" (Hegel, 1821, p. 7). Philosophy has some value if used retrospectively, as a tool for understanding the past, but it generally tells us little or nothing about the future. However, in the present case, current attempts to assimilate diseases to the etiological standpoint suggest that we are at a crisis, and many epidemiologists and even some philosophers have argued that this way of thinking has run its course (Broadbent, 2009). If there is to be further success in understanding disease, we may require a different model or at least a fundamental alteration of the current one. So, from this point of view, if one asks what progress are we now to expect in medicine, at least in this sense, and because of the limitations inherent in the etiological standpoint itself, the answer may be, *not much.* While I agree that we may be at a crisis point, I am less pessimistic about the future of the etiological standpoint than others seem to be; perhaps the demise of this way of thinking is neither imminent nor inevitable.

I

In chapter 7, we discussed, briefly, Edwin Klebs's *Grundversuche*. As Klebs made clear, the *Grundversuche* were to be used in conjunction with a set of causal criteria by means of which one could establish which specific bacterium causes a particular disease. So what are the causal criteria that must be satisfied once the *Grundversuche* are in place? Klebs's criteria involved isolating a particular form of bacterium from a diseased person or animal, cultivating it in an inert medium, and, under appropriate laboratory conditions, reproducing the disease by introducing organisms of that sort into susceptible animals.

Shortly after publication of the *Grundversuche*, Robert Koch adopted Klebs's causal criteria in his own research (Carter, 1985b); partly because these criteria became famous through Koch's celebrated papers on tuberculosis, the criteria are now called Koch's Postulates. Koch used the postulates as a central part of the research strategy that he called the *etiological standpoint* (Koch, 1901, p. 905). Like his friend Klebs, Koch was more interested in conducting research than in describing his own methods, so his account of the etiological standpoint, like Klebs's discussion of the *Grundversuche*, leaves much to be desired. However, from his publications, one can see how the etiological standpoint works at least in respect to bacterial diseases (Carter, 2003, pp. 129–46). With a theory in place (e.g., a set of laws more or less like Klebs's *Grundversuche*) and given a new disease, one identifies a bacterium that satisfies the causal criteria. One then recharacterizes the disease as infestation by that particular organism. This linguistic move is a crucial step: it creates a new disease, albeit one called by the same name as the given disease and sharing most of its instances. By definition, the new disease has a universal and necessary cause. The existence of such a cause, which must now, by definition, be present in every case of the disease, provides a basis for systematic explanations of disease phenomena and can sometimes suggest effective prophylactic and therapeutic strategies. As we have seen, without the new definition, as long as a disease is characterized symptomatically, identifying systematic explanations and reliable strategies for control is much more difficult if not impossible. Thus, the possibility of causal concepts of disease is a prerequisite or precondition that underlies the whole etiological standpoint.

In the 1880s and 1890s, Koch, Louis Pasteur, their students, and numerous other researchers identified various bacterial diseases. At almost the same time, protozoa were identified as causes of malaria, Texas fever, and of a few other diseases, and continuing on into the early decades of the twentieth century, a wide range of diseases were attributed to what were initially called filterable viruses (Carter, 2003, pp. 162–78). Of course, these causal agents were different from bacteria, and they required slightly different causal criteria and theories of disease—for one thing, being, for the most part, obligate and species-specific parasites, neither protozoa nor viruses could be grown in inert media or inoculated into test animals as required by the Postulates. However, the required modifications were relatively minor, and these diseases were assimilated to the etiological standpoint without much effort.

To a large extent, the etiological standpoint grew from work on bacterial and viral diseases. But it was clear from the outset that this approach was not limited to these diseases. A few years after Koch's famous papers on tuberculosis, Adolf von Strümpell, a Viennese psychologist, observed that "the scientific treatment of the etiology of diseases constitutes the most characteristic thrust of modern pathology; . . . and the secure establishment of the theory of organized, externally invading disease agents is until now the most beautiful and important achievement of this effort" (Strümpell, 1884, p. 2). Strümpell distinguished clearly between scientific etiology in general and work on the infectious diseases, which he described as "until now [scientific etiology's] most . . . important achievement." Implicit in this distinction is the recognition that noninfectious etiologies could be approached in the same way and could also yield impressive results. The clear assumption was that new theories would arise that would define new noninfectious kinds of causes, and, as one looks at medical research toward the end of the nineteenth century, that is precisely what one finds.

During the 1880s, Strümpell and P.J. Möbius argued that the psychological disorders were due to what they called pathogenic ideas—ideas that could, in a figurative sense, invade a human psyche, much like bacteria invading a body, and produce disease symptoms (Carter, 2003, pp. 147–61). This was referred to as the ideational theory of disease. This theory and the etiological standpoint in general were the model for Freud's early attempts to characterize hysteria and the anxiety neuroses in terms of prepubescent experiences or fantasies. The ideational theory of disease remains plausible and suggestive, and it contributed directly to the so-called talking cures that are still central to much of psychotherapy. However, the ideational theory has provided few empirically verifiable explanations, and it has often been dismissed as empty question begging. Yet it was probably the first attempt to assimilate a range of noninfectious diseases to the etiological standpoint. Other monocausal theories of disease, which arose at about the same time and which were also inspired by the etiological standpoint, have proven more effective.

Also beginning in the 1880s and continuing into the first decades of the twentieth century, research on beriberi culminated in the deficiency theory of disease, which explained not only beriberi, but scurvy, pellagra, and a few other disorders. This theory, with its associated causal criteria, was first articulated in a 1912 paper by Casimir Funk. While Funk did not state, concisely, a theory or causal criteria, after the manner of Klebs's *Grundversuche* or the Postulates, many of the elements essential for a theory of disease are explicit in his paper: Funk assumed (1) that a wide range of diseases are caused by deficiencies of what he initially referred to as *vitamines*, (2) that distinguishable diseases are caused by deficiencies of chemically distinguishable vitamines, (3) that the human body is incapable of producing its own adequate supplies of vitamines, and (4) that a normal balanced diet provides an ample supply of these elements. These assumptions resemble and more or less parallel the *Grundversuche*. As I have argued elsewhere, the etiological standpoint was the model for the elaboration of the deficiency theory of disease (Carter, 2003, pp. 179–95).

As we have seen in chapter 7, between 1866 and 1956, a number of genetic abnormalities were assimilated to the etiological standpoint. Like Funk's early paper on the deficiency diseases, Adrien Bleyer's original paper proposing that Down syndrome was a chromosomal nondisjunction, which we considered in chapter 7, reveals the outlines of a monocausal theory that could easily be expanded to accommodate many of these more recently discovered anomalies.

The most recently identified class of causes are prions that may account for the transmissible spongiform encephalopathies and, possibly, for a few other disorders such as sporadic fatal insomnia. While some researchers continue to argue that these disorders result ultimately from viruses or bacteria, most seem currently to accept the idea that prions do not depend on microorganisms. According to the dominant point of view, a prion is simply a misfolded protein molecule whose presence may launch a cascade of other similarly misformed molecules.

Given a sufficient number of prions, symptoms appear and, ultimately, the victim may succumb. If prions are introduced into a susceptible host by the consumption of infected tissues or by blood transfusions, for example, the disease may spread. Once again, one could formulate an explicit and general theory to account for this family of disorders as well as specific causal criteria by means of which to prove causal connections.

So far I have summarized what appears to be indisputable progress in medicine—progress in understanding and, in some cases, in controlling diseases. This progress resulted from following a certain approach, an approach that Koch called the etiological standpoint. Central to this approach are the adoption of monocausal theories of disease, the identification of suitable causal criteria, and the recharacterization of diseases so that each disease has a cause that is necessary and, therefore, universal. While medical researchers have given some attention to the causal criteria (often in the context of disputes over whether, in a particular case, the criteria have been satisfied), neither the *theories*, which are mostly implicit, nor the *strategy* of redefining diseases in terms of causes has received significant philosophical or historical scrutiny. However, each of these elements is crucial, and much of what counts as medical progress has come directly or indirectly from their use. So what basis can there be for doubting that this kind of progress will continue?

II

In a recent paper, Alex Broadbent describes what looks like a crisis in contemporary epidemiology: epidemiologists appear to have lost confidence in the monocausal model (Broadbent, 2009). As Broadbent explains, the problem has arisen because certain prominent classes of diseases defy every attempt at assimilation to this way of thinking (Broadbent, 2009, p. 302). These diseases, which can be loosely characterized as chronic noncommunicable diseases, include most forms of cancer, the autoimmune degenerative diseases such as rheumatoid arthritis, Crohn's disease, irritable bowel syndrome, pancreatitis, and other endocrinopathies, and various other disorders such as autism, Alzheimer's, diabetes, fibromyalgia, chronic fatigue syndrome, and many, many more. In each case, rather than a single cause in terms of which a disease can be characterized, research yields only statistical evidence of the etiological role both of genetic and of diverse environmental factors. In short, for each disease, one finds only a plurality

139

of unrelated risk factors. The analogy with early nineteenth-century causal thinking is obvious; indeed, Broadbent points out that the main difference between modern epidemiology and early nineteenth-century multifactorial accounts is that "modern epidemiology is able to supply more precise lists of causal factors, since it has more advanced statistical and experimental techniques" (Broadbent, 2009, p. 307). Of course, the appeal to multiple causes is not in itself unusual or problematic: in one sense, medicine has never abandoned this way of thinking, not even in regard to paradigmatic monocausal diseases like tuberculosis or beriberi. Even in such cases what is usually identified as *the* cause is necessary but not sufficient to explain the onset of any particular disease episode; and, of course, even this necessity is achieved not so much by discovery as by linguistic means—by re-characterizing a disease in terms of the purported cause. To explain any particular instance of tuberculosis or beriberi, for example, one must appeal to vague and imperfectly understood conditions that may contribute in some way or other to what is called *susceptibility*, and under this heading, one finds a plurality of possible risk factors. The difference is, in contrast to diseases like tuberculosis or beriberi, for chronic noncommunicable diseases, there is, at present, no single factor whose identification seems to provide a basis for explanation and control. Epidemiologists seem to have become more and more convinced that this lack is irremediable, and the monocausal model is now viewed with deep and widespread skepticism. As Broadbent points out, "A view of disease as multifactorial now dominates epidemiology" (Broadbent, 2009, p. 302).

However, as Broadbent recognizes, the resurgence of a multifactorial approach is hardly a welcome development, and his concern seems exactly right. "Risk factors," he points out, "are mere correlations" so while "identifying risk factors can be useful for devising public health interventions, . . . no catalogue of the risk factors for [a] disease will entail a general explanation of that disease, no matter how thorough the catalogue is" (Broadbent, 2009, p. 307). Yet, as Broadbent observes, we expect science to provide general explanations, and, indeed, explanations exactly of the sort that the etiological standpoint has so spectacularly generated for more than a century. So what is to be done? Can epidemiology continue to provide general explanations such as we have come to expect? Broadbent sees little hope in resuscitating the monocausal model. Not only is it awash in a sea of anomalies that it seems unable to assimilate, but he finds it to be philosophically defective as well. So, as a way forward, he proposes a different approach, one that he calls the contrastive model. No doubt this model warrants careful attention—it may just be the way of the future. However, while I agree with Broadbent's analysis of the current crisis and also with his criticism of the multifactorial approach, I am not persuaded by his objections to the monocausal model. I am not convinced that this way of thinking about diseases is no longer viable.

So what are the objections to the monocausal model? Broadbent identifies four. The *first*, which he regards as "the most obvious," is that "the monocausal model provides no justification for its restriction on the number of causes by which a disease may be defined . . .. To take a simple example," he continues, "swine influenza as it occurs naturally is caused by the synergistic action of a bacterium and a virus, . . . instances of the virus may exist in healthy animals without the bacteria, and vice versa" (Broadbent, 2009, p. 304). But I see this as no problem at all. The monocausal model imposes no restriction whatsoever on the number of causes by which a disease can be defined: let the virologists classify swine influenza as viral and let the bacteriologists classify it as bacterial. For that matter, since, at least in pigs, the disease seems to occur most often in conjunction with certain nutritional abnormalities, let animal nutritionists classify it as a monocausal nutritional disorder. And, since the disease almost certainly involves genetic dispositions, it can also be classified as genetic. Conceivably, the disease could also correlate with exposure to certain environmental toxins—such exposure could also be a risk factor. If so, this could provide yet a further way of classifying the disorder. Which classification is correct? Perhaps all are equally correct. From a theoretical point of view, one would probably favor whichever account seems to have the greatest explanatory power. From a practical perspective, if one or another way of classifying provides the most effective tools for control, that way will probably be adopted. However, neither from a theoretical nor from a practical point of view is there anything in the monocausal model that precludes the possibility of employing multiple, overlapping, monocausal explanations of a single disease. In each such explanation, one factor is sought in terms of which the disease is classified, explained, and attacked; of course, these different schemes will be inconsistent with one another, but that poses no problem nor does it undermine the fact that each single scheme is monocausal. Presumably, neither in offering explanations nor in seeking control would a single person adopt more than one scheme at a given time, but there is no reason why, for different purposes, the same person couldn't adopt different, inconsistent, accounts of the disease at different times. Such a plurality of points of view is the normal fare in science—this is why, as Norwood Russell Hansen helped us understand decades ago, one can assume that gasses are continuous while doing acoustics and yet assume that they are composed of discrete particles while working out issues involving heat and pressure (Hansen, 1963). Why should medicine be denied the same flexibility? The monocausal model is not incompatible with this kind of pluralism. Of course, I very much doubt that the original framers of the etiological standpoint thought in these terms, but what they may have thought should certainly not restrict our use of the model today.

Broadbent's *second* objection to the monocausal model is that, while it requires us to reclassify diseases, it "does not tell us how to do this . . . [and] there will generally be more than one [possible] reclassification of symptomatically grouped illnesses" (Broadbent, 2009, p. 305). As an example, he cites tuberculosis for which, by definition, tubercle bacilli are necessary. But, Broadbent points out, "A lack of inherited immunity is also necessary." So he asks, "What is to stop us [from] saying 'tuberculosis is inherited,' and defining tuberculosis as a hereditary vulnerability to an organism that occurs in our environment?" (Broadbent, 2009, p. 305). The answer, of course, is that nothing can or should prevent us from doing so. We can adopt *both* positions, although one would probably not apply them both simultaneously. If, on some occasion, there are theoretical or practical reasons for preferring one classification over the other, so be it; in the absence of such reasons, the choice may be arbitrary. But having made the choice on one occasion by, say, thinking of tuberculosis as hereditary, there is nothing to prevent us, on another occasion, from thinking of it as infectious. Indeed, it may even prove useful to alternate between these and even other points of view. Each way of thinking will entail its own system of analogies and connections: while thinking of tuberculosis as hereditary, we may notice certain relations to other inherited qualities (gender or blood type, perhaps) or to other diseases that also involve hereditary dispositions, whereas, while we think of it as infectious or dietary, we may become aware of yet other analogies. But this is hardly a problem—it may be a great advantage, both theoretically and practically. The more points of view we can adopt—the more schemes for classifying we can invoke—the better.

A *third* objection is that "the monocausal model might be thought to represent a sort of biological chauvinism: a refusal to countenance causes of ill health that are not biological" (Broadbent, 2009, p. 305). From what I have said so far, my response is probably obvious: bring on other monocauses and the new classifications they entail—the more the better. Broadbent, here following Katherine Angel, is concerned that "social, economic and psychological causes are, prima facie, very unlikely to display the sort of universality and uniformity which would allow them to qualify as causes for diseases on the monocausal model" (Broadbent, 2009, p. 305). But I don't see why—for any risk factor, universality can be achieved by mere definition, and, indeed, it seems quite plausible that the psychological issues such as those Angel and Broadbent are concerned should not be ignored—maybe even what Strümpell and Möbius called pathogenic ideas—could be involved in many diseases. As Kant helped us understand, the cause of any event is usually not another event but rather an open-ended set of conditions that precede or are simultaneous with that event. When we choose to identify one of these conditions as *the cause* of some event, it is usually because that single condition promises to give us particular understanding of or control over the event. This isn't so much a matter of metaphysics as of practicality, and I see no reason why the cause of a particular event could not be identified differently in different contexts and for different purposes especially by different persons who are particularly qualified to invoke different explanatory schemes or means of control.

A final objection is that the monocausal model "does not readily account for cases where a disease is present in a healthy individual. Yet this is nearly ubiquitous. Almost every disease is such that its cause may be present without causing the disease" (Broadbent, 2009, p. 305). In fact, the monocausal model seldom advances causes as being both necessary and sufficient. Indeed, adoption of monocausal character-izations created, for the first time in history, the very possibility of clinically inapparent and of psychosomatic disease episodes; in each of these situations, the disease itself is split apart from its symptoms, and both concepts (disease without symptoms and symptoms without disease) may be useful in both conceptual or practical ways. So this capacity, which may be impossible so long as we restrict our thinking to risk factors, can be seen as a strength of the monocausal model, and I'm far from regarding it as a problem. But it does point up another aspect of the whole issue of disease explanations to which I now turn.

Broadbent contrasts what he calls general and particular explanations. "A general explanation is one which holds for all the events in a given class, while a particular explanation says why some particular event or events occurred" (Broadbent, 2009, p. 306). Broadbent observes that "science gives both general and particular explanations: we can have a scientific explanation for the dropping of a single penny as well as for the falling of objects everywhere" (Broadbent, 2009, p. 307). He also acknowledges, as we have already noted, that the monocausal model provides general explanations. However, so far, neither the monocausal nor the multifactorial model provides much help when it comes to explaining individual disease episodes: so far, in explaining particular cases of disease, both approaches leave us with the hopelessly vague and almost always circular concept of susceptibility. Yet here a pluralistic monocausal model may offer some hope.

As I have explained, the monocausal model allows for a variety of different and inconsistent ways of defining and classifying; I've said that theoretical or practical considerations may incline us to move between these different schemes for defining and classifying—depending on the circumstances, we adopt now one and now another definition. Suppose we visualize these independent and inconsistent monocausal schemes as semitransparent grids that overlie the range of all disease episodes. Within any one grid, many disease episodes are classified according to the scheme in some particular grid or other. In some of the grids, the classification will be in terms of infective agents, in others in terms of dietary, environmental, hereditary, or even psychological factors, and perhaps some of these can be further divided into still more specific grids as, for example, the infectious grid can be divided into bacterial, viral, and other grids. Yet each grid, by itself, is monocausal. Given a single disease episode, say a case of swine influenza, looking horizontally, within any single grid, that episode would be classified in one way or another as determined by the nature of that particular grid; within a different grid, it will be classified differently. In some grids, for example, in a psychological grid, swine influenza may not appear at all. But what if we now look *vertically* at this one episode of swine influenza; what if we now gaze down through the whole collection of superimposed grids. We would see the single episode of swine influenza simultaneously within various monocausal schemes for classifying. On one grid, we see it classified as a combination of certain nutritional deficiencies, on another, as a certain gene pattern where it may be linked with other disease episodes that may not even be symptomatically similar, on the environmental toxin grid it may be linked up with yet other cases of disease, on the virus and bacterial grids it is classified still differently. In principle, if we have enough grids that take account of enough factors, the collection of all these factors could turn out to be jointly sufficient for that particular disease episode. The vague concept of susceptibility, which is inescapable so long as one's attention is focused horizontally, within any one grid, is now replaced by the combination of factors that may, jointly, completely explain that one disease episode. In short, the intersection of the various general explanations provided by the different and inconsistent monocausal models could yield a complete and sufficient explanation for that one particular event. In this way, our plurality of monocausal models may provide a complete and perfect understanding of how one person becomes diseased while another person can carry tubercle bacilli without showing any symptoms. Given this way of approaching disease explanations, medical science may ultimately provide both general and particular explanations exactly as Broadbent requires.

So, is this what the future of epidemiology holds? I believe it may be the ideal. Will that ideal ever be realized? Perhaps. There may be progress within many of the explanatory grids currently in use, especially within those that are currently relatively undeveloped, and here genetic and molecular medicine seem particularly promising. Alternatively, entirely new grids may be discovered. So multiple monocauses may still offer hope for the etiological standpoint. Of course, it could happen that this ideal is never to be realized. It may be that our quest for such explanations will simply never end. There may be diseases for which the identification of causes is impossible, and if so, this impossibility could be a matter of principle or merely a practical consequence of our own limitations. On analogy with what we have learned about quantum physics, there could be disease episodes that have no sufficient causes—they simply happen. This seems especially plausible given that all diseases must, ultimately, involve changes on a molecular level. This could mean that, finally, for some diseases, there is nothing beyond risk factors. Alternatively, there could be cases of illness that could, in principle, be completely explained, but for which identifying all the causes involved would require more intellectual, financial, and/or temporal assets than the human species will ever have at its disposal—in short, there could be diseases, maybe whole classes of them, with causes that we are simply not smart enough ever to identify. These are the kinds of problems that may ultimately impose bounds on the etiological standpoint and limit epidemiology to a disjoint collection of general explanations for a few isolated diseases and to risk factors for all the rest. And, of course, if there are such limits, we are unlikely ever to know that for sure, and so we may spend the rest of our time on earth looking for ways to fill the gaps without ever knowing with certainty whether the quest can, in principle, be completed. Ultimately, from an omniscient point of view, the epidemiologists' skepticism of the monocausal model may be entirely correct. In the meantime, I am not persuaded that there are sufficient reasons, just yet, for giving up on a model that has been so successful until now.

So what progress are we now to expect in medicine? Does the current crisis show that we are approaching the absolute limits of the scientific understanding of disease? Or is there a way forward? If there is to be progress, what will it involve? Contrastive models of disease causation? Pluralities of overlapping layers of monocauses? Or ways of thinking that are altogether different and so alien and strange as to be completely beyond any current philosophical speculation? In quite a different context, Karl Marx once observed that it is not for the philosophers to dictate recipes for the cook shops of the future. In the current situation, that kind of modesty, so uncharacteristic of Marx, seems to me entirely appropriate. So what progress are we now to expect in medicine? Only future science will tell; in the meantime, we can only wait and wash (Lumpe, 1850, p. 398).

References

Abernethy, Mr. (1824), "Introductory Surgical and Medical Lectures Delivered in London in the Month of October 1824," *Lancet*, 3:5–13.

Ackerknecht, Erwin H. (1946), "Natural Diseases and Rational Treatment in Primitive Medicine," *Bulletin of the History of Medicine*, 19:467–97.

Agassi, Joseph (1969), "The Concept of Scientific theory as Illustrated in the Practice of Bloodletting," *Medical Opinion*, 5:157–69.

Alison, William P. (1850), "Notice of Cases of Pleurisy and Pneumonia in the Clinical Wards of the Royal Infirmary in Summer 1850," *Monthly Journal of Medical Science*, 11:157–72.

Alison, William P. (1852), "Cases Illustrating the Asthenic Form of Internal Inflammations now Common in the Country," *Monthly Journal of Medical Science*, 15:493–507.

Alison, William P. (1855–6), "Reflections on the Results of Experience as to the Symptoms of Internal Inflammations, and the Effects of Bloodletting, during the last Forty Years," *Edinburgh Medical Journal*, 1: 769–88.

Alison, William P. (1856–7a), Discussion following lecture by John H. Bennett, "Observations on the Results of an Advanced Diagnosis and Pathology Applied to the Management of Internal Inflammations, Compared with the Effects of a Former Antiphlogistic Treatment, and Especially of Bloodletting," *Edinburgh Medical Journal*, 2:857–58.

Alison, William P. (1856–7b), "Reply to Dr. Bennett's Observations on the Results of an Advanced Diagnosis and Pathology in the Treatment of Internal Inflammations, Compared with the Effects of a Former Antiphlogistic Treatment, and Especially of Bloodletting," *Edinburgh Medical Journal*, 2:971–95, 1044–52.

Andral, Gabriel (1832–3), "Hydrophobia," *Lancet*, 1:806–08.

Armstrong, J. (1825), "From Lectures on the Principles and Practice of Physic, Lecture 27," *Lancet*, 7:261–66.

Ashwell, Samuel (1852), "A Practical Treatise on the Diseases Peculiar to Women," *Edinburgh Medical and Surgical Journal*, 77:417–50.

A.Z. (1827), Letter to the Editor, *Lancet*, xi:346.

Bardsley, James L. (1849), "Diabetes," in Forbes, Tweedie, and Conolly, 1:606–25.

Barlow, Edward (1849a), "Education (Physical)," in Forbes, Tweedy, and Conolly, 1:750–65.

Barlow, Edward (1849b), "Plethora," in Forbes, Tweedy, and Conolly, 3:553–74.

Bedford, G. S. (1868), *The Principles and Practice of Obstetrics*, 4th ed., New York, NY: William Wood.

Benedek, István (1983), *Ignaz Philipp Semmelweis*, Vienna, Austria: Hermann Böhlas.

Bennett, John H. (1855), *The Present State of the theory and Practice of Medicine*, Edinburgh, Scotland: Sutherland and Knox.

Bennett, John H. (1856–7a), "Observations on the Results of an Advanced Diagnosis and Pathology Applied to the Management of Internal Inflammations, Compared with the Effects of a Former Antiphlogistic Treatment, and Especially of Bloodletting," *Edinburgh Medical Journal*, 2:769–96.

Bennett, John H. (1856–7b), "A Reply to the Preceding Paper of Dr. Alison," *Edinburgh Medical Journal*, 2:995–1000.

Bennett, John H. (1856–7c), "A Reply to the Previous Note of Dr. Watson," *Edinburgh Medical Journal*, 2:1088–92.

Berman, Alex (1978), "The Heroic Approach in 19th Century Therapeutics," in Judith Walzer Leavitt and Ronald L. Numbers (Eds.), *Sickness and Health in America*, Madison, WI: University of Wisconsin Press.

Bettelheim, Bruno (1962) *Symbolic Wounds*, New York, NY: Collier Books.

Bleyer, Adrien (1934), "Indications That Mongoloid Imbecility Is a Gametic Mutation of Degressive Type," *American Journal of Diseases of Childhood*, 47:342–48.

Blundell, J. (1828), "Lectures on the Theory and Practice of Midwifery," *Lancet*, 9:577–83.

Boehr, Max (1868), "Ueber die Infectionstheorie des Puerperalfiebers und ihre Consequenzen für die Sanitäts-Polizei," *Monatsschrift für Geburtskunde und Frauenkrankheiten*, 32:401–33.

Brain, Peter (1986), *Galen on Bloodletting*, Cambridge: Cambridge University Press.

Broadbent, Alex (2009), "Causation and Models of Disease in Epidemiology," *Studies in the History and Philosophy of the Biological and Biomedical Sciences*, 40:302–11.

Brown, Joseph (1849), "Contagion," in Forbes, Tweedie, and Conolly, 1:500–05.

Brown, William (1818), "Observations on Bloodletting from the Hemorrhoidal Veins," *Edinburgh Medical and Surgical Journal*, 14:136–41.

Bryan, Leon S, Jr., 1964, "Bloodletting in American Medicine, 1830–1892," *Bulletin of the History of Medicine*, 5:516–29.

Buchan, William, 1779, *Domestic Medicine or a Treatise on the Prevention and Cure of Disease*, 6th ed., London: W. Straham.

Carter, K. Codell (1982) "On the Decline of Bloodletting in Nineteenth Century Medicine," *The Journal of Psychoanalytic Anthropology*, 5:219–34.

Carter, K. Codell (1985a), "Ignaz Semmelweis, Carl Mayrhofer, and the Rise of Germ Theory," *Medical History*, 29:33–53.

Carter, K. Codell (1985b), "Koch's Postulates in Relation to the Work of Jacob Henle and Edwin Klebs," *Medical History*, 29:353–74.

Carter, K. Codell (1991), "Causes of Disease and Death in the Babylonian Talmud," *Medizin-historisches Journal*, 26:94–104.

Carter, K. Codell (1993), "The Concept of Quackery in Early Nineteenth Century British Medical Periodicals," *The Journal of Medical Humanities*, 14:89–97.

Carter, K. Codell (2001), "Leechcraft in Nineteenth Century British Medicine," *Journal of the Royal Society of Medicine*, 94:38–42.

Carter, K. Codell (2002), "Early Conjectures that Down Syndrome Is Caused by Chromosomal Nondisjunction," *Bulletin of the History of Medicine*, 76:528–63.

Carter, K. Codell (2003), *The Rise of Causal Concepts of Disease*, Aldershot, England: Ashgate Publishing Limited.

Carter, K. Codell (2005), *A First Course in Logic*, New York, NY: Pearson.

Carter, K. Codell (2010), "Change of Type as an Explanation for the Decline of Therapeutic Bloodletting," *Studies in the History and Philosophy of Biological and Biomedical Sciences*, 41:1–11.

Carter, K. Codell and Barbara R. Carter (1994), *Childbed Fever: A Scientific Biography of Ignaz Semmelweis*, Westport, CT: Greenwood Press (paperback edition with some minor changes (2005) Transaction Publishers).

Carter, K. Codell, Scott Abbott, and James L. Siebach (1995), "Five Documents Relating to the Final Illness and Death of Ignaz Semmelweis," *Bulletin of the History of Medicine*, 69:255–70.

Castiglioni, Arturo (1947), *A History of Medicine*, 2nd ed., E. B. Krumbhaar (trans.), New York, NY: Alfred A. Knopf.

Chomel, M. (1838), "Etiologie," in Adelon, *Dictionnaire de médecine*, 12:415–25.

Christison, R. (1857–8), "On the Changes Which Have Taken Place in the Constitution of Fevers and Inflammations," *Edinburgh Medical Journal*, 3:577–95.

Clutterbuck, H. (1826), "Lectures on the Theory and Practice of Physic: Lecture XX," *Lancet*, 10:7–12.

Clutterbuck, H. (1838a), "Lectures on Bloodletting: Lecture III," *London Medical Gazette*, 2:166–70.

Clutterbuck, H. (1838b), "Lectures on Bloodletting: Lecture IV," *London Medical Gazette*, 2:209–16.

Conrad, Peter and Joseph W. Schneider (1980), *Deviance and Medicalization: From Badness to Sickness*, St. Louis, MO: C. V. Mosby Company.

Connor, Michael and Malcolm Ferguson-Smith (1997), *Essential Medical Genetics*, 5th ed., Oxford, England: Blackwell Science.

Conolly, John (1849), "Disease," in Forbes, Tweedie, and Conolly, 1:674–89.

Cooper, Astley (1823), "Lectures on Irritation and Inflammation," *Lancet*, i:322.

Cooper, Astley (1823–4), "Medical Lectures," *Lancet*, i:115.

Crampton, Philip (1822), "On the Application of Leeches to Internal Surfaces," *Dublin Hospital Reports*, 3:223–30.

Crawford, Adair (1849), "Convulsions," in Forbes, Tweedy, and Conolly, 1:508–19.

Cumin, William (1849), "Scrofula," in Forbes, Tweedie, and Conolly, 4:125–45.

Cumming, W. (1853), "General Bloodletting, With Illustrative Cases," *Lancet*, 62:242–45.

Cyclops (1840–1), "Letter to the Editor," *Lancet*, i:102.

Darwell, John (1849), "Anasarca," in Forbes, Tweedy, and Conolly, 1:95–103.

DeLacy, Margaret (1989), "Puerperal Fever in Eighteenth-Century Britain," *Bulletin of the History of Medicine*, 63:521–56.

Delpech, Jacques Mathieu (1825), "Case of a Wound of the Right Carotid Artery," *Lancet*, 6:210–13.

Dendy, Walter C. (1840–1), "Letter to the Editor," *Lancet*, 1840–1, i:165.

De Vos, George A. (1975), "The Dangers of Pure Theory in Social Anthropology," *Ethos*, 3:77–91.

Douglas, Mary (1975), *Implicit Meanings*, London: Routledge & Kegan Paul.

Down, John Langdon (1866), "Ethnic Classification of Idiots," *London Hospital Clinical Lectures and Reports*, 3:259–62; reprinted in John Landgon Down, *On Some of the Mental Affections of Childhood and Youth* (1887), London: Churchill, pp. 210–17.

Dunn, Peter M. (2000), "Dr. William Buchan (1729–1805) and his *Domestic Medicine*," *Archive of Diseases of Children and Fetal and Neonatal Education*, 83:F71–F73.

Easton, J. A. (1857–8), "Clinical Lecture on Pneumonia," *Edinburgh Medical Journal*, 3:703–12.

Editor (1824), "Documents Relative to the History of the Malignant Puerperal Fever Which Prevailed in the Lying-in Institution in Vienna from the Beginning of August to the middle of November 1819," *Edinburgh Medical and Surgical Journal*, 22:83–91.

Editor's Note (1799), *London Medical Journal*, i:337.

Editor's Note (1802), *London Medical Journal*, 7:397f.

Editor's Note (1810), *London Medical Journal*, 23:64.

Editor's Note (1821), *Medical Repository*, 15:358.

Editor's Note (1823), *Lancet*, i:664.

Editor's Note (1824), *Medical Repository*, 2:166–72.

Editor's Note (1827–8), *Lancet*, ii:14.

Editor's Note (1828–9), "Pregnancy after Excision of the Os Uteri," *Lancet*, ii:192.

Editor's Note (1829–30), *Lancet*, ii:470.

Editor's Note (1835–6), *Lancet*, ii:57.

Editor's Note (1838–9a), *Lancet*, i:112.

Editor's Note (1838–9b), *Lancet*, ii:874.

Editor's Note (1839–40), *Lancet*, ii:877.

Editor's Note (1840–1), *Lancet*, ii:57.

Editor's Note (1846), *Lancet*, i:191.

Editor's Note (1843–4), *Lancet*, i:424.

Editor's Note (1845), Lancet, ii:629.

Editor's Notes (1823), *Lancet*, i:24, 38, 55, 94, 257.

Editor's Notes (1840–1), *Lancet*, i:61f, 132, 421, 711.

Editor's Notes (1846), *Lancet*, i:191, 226, 368.

Editor's Review (1829–30), *Lancet*, ii:709.

Editor's Review (1842-3), "Bloodletting," *Lancet*, ii:838.

Editor's Review (1854), *Lancet*, ii:199.

Eliot, George (1984), *Middlemarch*, London: Penguin; originally published 1871–2.

Elliotson, John (1844), *Principles and Practice of Medicine*, 2nd ed., London: Carey and Hart.

Epler, D. C. Jr. (1980), "Bloodletting in Early Chinese Medicine and its Relation to the Origin of Acupuncture," *Bulletin of the History of Medicine*, 54:337–67.

Evans-Pritchard, E. E. (1976), *Witchcraft, Oracles, and Magic among the Azende*, Abridged Ed., Oxford: Oxford University Press.

Fischel, Wilhelm (1882), "Zur Therapie der puerperalen Sepsis," *Archiv für Gynaekologie*, 20:1–70.

Flaubert, Gustave (1950), *Madame Bovary*, London: Penguin Books.

Flemming, Percy (1957), "Medical Aspects of the Mediaeval Monastery in England," in Zachary Cope (Ed.), *Sidelights on the History of Medicine*, London: Butterworth and Company.

Forbes, John (1849), "Angina Pectoris," in Forbes, Tweedie, and Conolly, 1:103–17.

Forbes, John, Alexander Tweedie, and John Conolly (Eds.) (1849), *The Cyclopaedia of Practical Medicine*, revised with additions by Robley Dunglison, Philadelphia, PA: Lea and Blanchard.

Foster, George M. (1965), "Disease Etiologies in Non-Western Medical Systems," *American Anthropologist*, 78:773–82.

Foucault, Michel (1973), *The Birth of the Clinic*, New York, NY: Pantheon Books.

Frankfurt, H. A., John A. Wilson, and Thorkild Jacobsen (1949), *Before Philosophy*, London: Penguin Books.

Funk, Casimir, 1912, "The Etiology of the Deficiency Diseases," *Journal of State Medicine*, 20:341–68.

Gairdner, W. T. (1857–8), "Remarks on Dr. Bennett's Paper on Bloodletting and Antiphlogistic Treatment," *Edinburgh Medical Journal*, 3:197–232.

Gester (1847), "Das medicinische Wien," *Archiv für physiologische Heilkunde*, 6:320–29, 468–80.

Glick, Leonard B. (1967), "Medicine as an Ethnographic Category: The Gimi of the New Guinea Highlands," *Ethnology*, 6:31–56.

Goldie, George (1849), "Haematemesis," in Forbes, Tweedie, and Conolly, 2:357–62.

Gortvay, György and Imre Zoltán (1968), *Semmelweis: His Life and Work*, Budapest: Akadémiai Kiadó.

Grower, S. (1831–2) "Treatment of Puerperal Fever; Bloodletting by Leeches," *Lancet*, i:120.

Halbertsma, T. (1923), "Mongolism in One of Twins and the Etiology of Mongolism," *American Journal of Diseases of Children*, 25:350–53.

Haller, John S. (1982), *American Medicine in Transition, 1840–1910*, Illinois: University of Illinois.

Hansen, Norwood Russell (1963), *Patterns of Discovery*, Cambridge: Cambridge University Press.

Hegel, G. W. F. (1821), Preface to *Philosophy of Right*, Great Books of the Western World, Encyclopedia Britannica, Inc.

Henderson, George (1828–9), "Letter to the Editor," *Lancet*, ii:614–16.

Holmes, Oliver Wendell (1843), "The Contagiousness of Puerperal Fever," reprinted in *Medical Essays* (1883), Boston, MA: Houghton Mifflin.

Jacob, Arthur (1849), "Ophthalmia," Forbes, Tweedy, and Conolly, 3:413–36.
Jex-Blake, Sophia (1877), "Puerperal Fever: An Inquiry into Its Nature and Treatment," M.D. Dissertation, University of Bern.
King, Lester S. (1961), "The Bloodletting Controversy: A Study in the Scientific Method," *Bulletin of the History of Medicine*, 35:1–13.
King, Lester S. (1982), *Medical Thinking: A Historical Preface*, Princeton, NJ: Princeton University Press.
Klebs, Edwin (1875–6), "Beiträge zur Kenntniss der pathogenen Schistomyceten," *Archiv für experimentelle Pathologie und Pharmakologie*, 3:305–24, 4:107–36, 207–47, 374–77, 409–88.
Koch, Robert, 1901, "Massnahmen gegen die Pest," in J. Schwalbe (Ed.) 1912, *Gesammelte Werke von Robert Koch*, Leipzig: George Thieme, vol. 1, pp. 905–07.
Lagasquie, A. (1849), "Causes," in Jean Pierre Beaude (Ed.), *Dictionnaire de médecine usuelle à l'usaes des gens du mode*, 1:313, Paris: Didier.
Lakatos, Imre (1968), "Falsification and the Methodology of Scientific Research Programmes," in Imre Lakatos and Alan Musgrave (Eds.) (1974), *Criticism and the Growth of Knowledge*, Cambridge: Cambridge University Press, pp. 91–196.
Landau, L. (1875), "Das Puerperalfieber und die Gebärhäuser," *Berliner klinische Wochenschrift*, 12:150–52, 166–69.
Lavoisier, Antoine Laurent (1789), *Elements of Chemistry*, Great Books of the Western World, Encyclopaedia Britannica, Inc.
Law, Robert (1849), "Haemoptysis," in Forbes, Tweedy, and Connoly, 2:362–71.
Lawrence, W. (1825), "Lectures on the Anatomy, Physiology, and Diseases of the Eye," *Lancet*, 5:401–07.
Lawrence, W. (1827), "Extract from Mr. Lawrence's Introductory Lecture to the Spring Course of Surgery," *Lancet*, 7:629–34.
Lawrence, W. (1829–30), "Lectures on Surgery, Medical and Operative, Lecture IV: Inflammation," *Lancet*, i:137–41,169–74, 201–06, 265–71.
Leake, Chauncey D. (Ed.) (1927), *Percival's Medical Ethics*, Philadelphia, PA: Williams and Wilkins Company.
Lisfranc, M. (1833-4), "Diseases of the Uterus," *Lancet*, i:438.
Lisfranc, M. (1836), "Observations on Local and General Bloodletting," *London Medical Gazette*, 17:841–43.
Loudon, Irvine (1986), *Medical Care and the General Practitioner 1750–1850*, Oxford, England: Clarendon Press.
Loudon, Irvine (2000), *The Tragedy of Childbed Fever*, Oxford: Oxford University Press.
Louis, Pierre-Charles-Alexandre (1828), "Recherche sur les effets de la saignée dans plusieurs maladies inflammatoires," *Archives générales de médecin*, 18:321–36.
Lumpe, Eduard (1845), "Die Leistungen der neuesten Zeit in der Gynäkologie," *Zeitschruft der k. k.Gesellschaft der Aerzte zu Wien*, 1:341–71.
Lumpe, Eduard (1850), "Zur Theorie der Puerperalfieber," *Zeitschrift der k. k. Gesellschaft der Aerzte zu Wien*, 6:392–98.

Mann, Thomas (1936), "Freud und die Zukunft," *Thomas Mann Gesammelte Werke* (1960) 9:489.

Markham, William O. (1857), "Remarks on the Inflammation and Bloodletting Controversy," *Lancet*, 70:439–41, 465–67, 493–95, 515–17, 571–73, 595–97.

Markham, William O. (1866), *Bleeding and Change of Type of Diseases*, London: John Churchill & Sons.

McAdam, E. L., Jr. and George Milne (Eds.) (1965), *Johnson's Dictionary*, New York, NY: Modern Library.

McKendrick, N., J. Brewer, and J. H. Plumb (1982), *The Birth of a Consumer Society*, London: Europa.

McKeown, Thomas (1976), *The Modern Rise of Population*, London: Edward Arnold.

M.D. (1845), Letter to the Editor, *Lancet*, ii:629.

Miller, C. M. (1848), "On the Treatment of Puerperal Fever," *Lancet*, 2:262.

Niebyl, Peter H. (1977), "The English Bloodletting Revolution, or Modern Medicine before 1850," *Bulletin of the History of Medicine*, 51:464–83.

Osborne, J. (1833), "Observations on Local Bloodletting and Methods of Practicing It," *Dublin Journal of Medical and Chemical Science*, 3:334–42.

Oxtoby, David W. and Norman H. Nachtrieb (1990), *Principles of Modern Chemistry*, Saunders College Publishing.

Pasteur, Louis (1881), "Vaccination in Relation to Chicken-Cholera and Splenic Fever," reprinted in Vallery-Radot Pasteur (Ed.) (1922–39), *Oeuvres de Pasteur*, 7 vols, Paris, 6:370–78.

Pellegrino, Edmund D., (1983), "Hospitals as Moral Agents: Some Notes about Institutional Ethics," in Natalie Abrams and Michael D. Buckner (Eds.), *Medical Ethics*, Cambridge, MA: MIT Press.

Pelling, Margaret and Charles Webster (1979), "Medical Practitioners," in Charles Webster (Ed.), *Health, Medicine and Morality in the Sixteenth Century*, Cambridge: Cambridge University Press.

Pink Saucer and Blue Light (1840–1), "Letter to the Editor," *Lancet*, i:322–23.

Polunin, Ivan (1977), "Disease, Morbidity, and Mortality in China, India, and the Arab World," in Charles Leslie (Ed.), *Asian Medical Systems*, California: University of California.

Porter, Roy (1989), *Health for Sale, Quackery in England 1660–1850*, Manchester, UK: Manchester University Press.

Prichard, J. C. (1849a), "Hypochondriasis," in Forbes, Tweedy, and Conolly, 2:554–62.

Prichard, J. C. (1849b), "Insanity," in Forbes, Tweedy, and Connolly, 3:26–76.

r. (1882), [Obituary of Carl Mayrhofer], *Wiener medizinische Blätter*, 5:col. 725.

Rosenberg, Charles E. (1979), "The Therapeutic Revolution: Medicine, Meaning, and Social Change in Nineteenth-Century America," in Morris J. Vogel and Charles E. Rosenberg, (Eds.), *The Therapeutic Revolution: Essays in the Social History of American Medicine*, Philadelphia, PA: University of Pennsylvania Press.

Roser, W. (1867), "Zur Verständigung über den Pyämiebegriff," *Archiv für Heilkunde*, 8:15–24.

Scanzoni, Wilhelm Friedrich (1850), "[Review of Josef] Skoda, Ueber die von Dr. Semmelweis entdeckte wahre Ursche der in der Wiener Gebäranstalt ungewöhnlich häufig vorkommenden Erkrankungen der Wöchnerinen," *Vierteljahrschrift für das praktische Heilkunde, Literarische Anzeiger*, 26:25–33.
Schönlein, Johann Lucas (1832), *Allgemeine und specielle Pathologie und Therapie*, 1841, Litteratur-Compoir.
Semmelweis, Ignaz (1861), *The Etiology, Concept, and Prophylaxis of Childbed Fever*, K. Codell Carter, trans., 1983, Wisconsin: University of Wisconsin.
Shorter, Edward (1980), "Women's Diseases before 1900," in Mel Albin (Ed.), *New Directions in Psychohistory*, Lanham, MD: Lexington Books, pp. 183–208.
Simpson, Charles (1848), "Letter to the Editor," *Lancet*, ii:431.
Stephens, J. (1857–8), "Letter to the Editor," *Edinburgh Medical Journal*, 3:184–86.
Strümpell, Adolf von (1884), "Ueber die Ursachen der Erkrankungen des Nervensystems," *Deutsche Archiv für klinische Medizin*, 35:1–17.
Sutherland, G. A. (1899), "Mongolian Imbecility in Infants," *Practioner*, 63:632–42.
Symonds, J. A. (1849), "Tetanus," in Forbes, Tweedy, and Conolly, 4:364–76.
Taylor, F. Kräupl (1979), *The Concepts of Illness, Disease and Morbus*, Cambridge: Cambridge University Press.
Townsend, Richard (1849), "Apoplexy (Pulmonary)," in Forbes, Tweedy, and Conolly, 1:155–63.
Trousseau, A., (1835), "Croup," in Adelon, *Dictionnaire de médecine*, 9:334–401.
Turnbull, W. (1857–8), "Letter to the Editor," *Edinburgh Medical Journal*, 3:186–88.
Turner, Victor (1967), *The Forest of Symbols*, Ithaca, NY: Cornell University Press.
Tweedie, Alexander (1849a), "Erysipelas," in Forbes, Tweedie, and Conolly, 2:96–105.
Tweedie, Alexander (1849b), "Fever (Continued)," in Forbes, Tweedie, and Conolly, 2:153–201.
Tyrrell, F. (1824), "Report of Cases at St. Thomas's Hospital," *Lancet*, iv:223.
Van der Steen, Wim J. and Harmke Kamminga (1991), "Laws and Natural History in Biology," *British Journal of the Philosophy of Science*, 42:445–67.
Veit, A. C. G. (1867), *Krankheiten der weiblichen Geschlechtsorgane*, 2nd ed., Erlangen, Germany: Ferdinand Enke.
Virchow, Rudolf (1856), *Gesammelte Abhandlungen zur wissenschaftlichen Medicine*, Frankfurt am Main, Germany: Meidinger & Sohn & Company.
Waddy, J. M. (1845), "On Puerperal Fever," *Lancet*, 2:671f.
Wardrop, James (1833), "Lectures on Surgery, by Mr. Wardrop. The Diseases of the Sanguineous System," *Lancet*, 21:236–42.
Wardrop, James (1833–4), "On the Sanguineous System; Abstraction of Blood," *Lancet*, i:816–24.
Warner, John Harley (1980), "Therapeutic Explanation and the Edinburgh Bloodletting Controversy: Two Perspectives on the Medical Meaning of Science in the Mid-Nineteenth Century," *Medical History*, 24:241–58.

Watson, Thomas (1856–7), "Note to the Lecture on Bloodletting, Formerly Published," *Edinburgh Medical Journal*, 2:1084–88.

Watson, Thomas (1858), *Lectures on the Principles and Practice of Physic*, Philadelphia, PA: Blanchard and Lea.

Wertheimer, M. (1888), *Von dem Verhalten der Lochialsecretion zur Pathogenese des Kindbettfiebers*, Freiburg, Germany: H. M. Poppen & Sohn.

White, Anthony (1819), "A Case of Haemorrhage which Terminated Fatally from the Application of a Leech," *London Medical Repository*, 11:23–26.

White, Charles (1773), *A Treatise on the Management of Pregnant and Lying-in Women*, London: E. and C. Cilly.

Wilkinson, G. (1804), "Remarks on the Preservation and Management of Leeches," *London Medical and Physical Journal*, 12:485–96.

Wilkinson, G. (1848), "Medical News," *Lancet*, i:624.

Winckel, Franz Karl Ludwig Wilhelm (1866), *Die Pathologie und Therapie des Wochenbettes*, Berlin: Hirschwald.

Wittgenstein, Ludwig (1958), *The Blue and the Brown Books*, New York, NY: Harper Torchbooks.

Wootton, David (2007), *Bad Medicine: Doctors Doing Harm Since Hippocrates*, Oxford: Oxford University Press.

Index

For Product Safety Concerns and Information please contact our
EU representative GPSR@taylorandfrancis.com Taylor & Francis
Verlag GmbH, Kaufingerstraße 24, 80331 München, Germany